SOUMIA BENBERNOU
NABIL GHOMARI
Fouzia kambouche

MYASTHENIA GRAVIS, DIAGNOSTIC DIFFICULTIES AND INTENSIVE CARE MANAGEMENT

SOUMIA BENBERNOU
NABIL GHOMARI
Fouzia kambouche

MYASTHENIA GRAVIS, DIAGNOSTIC DIFFICULTIES AND INTENSIVE CARE MANAGEMENT

ScienciaScripts

Imprint

Cover image: www.ingimage.com

This book is a translation from the original published under ISBN 978-620-6-70251-1.

Publisher:
Sciencia Scripts
is a trademark of
Dodo Books Indian Ocean Ltd. and OmniScriptum S.R.L publishing group

120 High Road, East Finchley, London, N2 9ED, United Kingdom
Str. Armeneasca 28/1, office 1, Chisinau MD-2012, Republic of Moldova, Europe
Printed at: see last page
ISBN: 978-620-7-62679-3

CONTENTS

PART THEORETICAL

I.INTRODUCTION :

Myasthenia is a chronic, disabling disease whose lesion is located between the nerve and the muscle, at the neuromuscular junction [18], affecting the somatic nervous system and therefore only striated muscles [19].
The damage is not to the muscle, so it's not strictly speaking a myopathy.
The nerve no longer correctly transmits to the muscle the nervous excitation that triggers muscle contraction. The result is muscle weakness of varying intensity and duration. This weakness increases with effort or repetition of movement, and can lead to partial paralysis of the muscle(s) concerned [18].

Myasthenia is also an autoimmune disease, like lupus, rheumatoid arthritis or certain forms of insulin-dependent diabetes. These diseases are characterized by the destruction of certain body components by the immune system, which mistakenly recognizes them as foreign elements.
People with myasthenia produce anti-RACh antibodies against their own acetylcholine receptors (RACh). These antibodies, by binding to the post-synaptic acetylcholine receptors located in the motor plate, cause their destruction or block their function[18].
Without acetylcholine, the transmission of nerve impulses to the muscle is impaired: the muscle contracts less and tires.
85% of people with myasthenia have anti-acetylcholine receptor antibodies in their serum [18], whereas these have never been found in other neuromuscular disorders [20].

Considered an orphan disease, myasthenia has no cure but only a preventive treatment.

II. LITERATURE REVIEW :

II.1.HISTORY :

It is likely that Thomas Willis, describing fluctuating paralysis as "paralysiaspuria non habitualis" in 1672, gave the first known description of MG.
As Oostherhuis[21] recalls, the first significant observation was made in 1868 by Hérard, a physician at the Lariboisière hospital in Paris. He reported the story of a woman suffering from intermittent disorders of phonation, swallowing, oculomotricity and motor control of the limbs, which were aggravated by menstruation and emotions; the patient died of acute respiratory failure.
This observation thus predates those of Erb and Goldflam.
Erb in 1879 and Goldflam in 1893 observed fluctuating symptoms, selective eye muscle involvement and worsening during the day.
In 1895, Jolly had the double merit of proposing the name "myasthenia gravispseudo paralytica" and demonstrating the exhaustion of muscular contraction under the effect of electrical stimulation.in 1901, Laquer and Weigert reported the association of thymoma-MG.in 1905, Buzzard, at the autopsy of a myasthenic, noted the existence of lymphophorragia in the muscles and lymphoid hyperplasia of the thymus.
In 1934, Mary Walker, struck by the similarity of the signs ofcurare intoxication and MG, advocated the use of physostigmine and then Prostigmine.the same year, Dale and Feldberg discovered that ACh was released at the neuromuscular junction.

In 1939, Blalock et al. reported the favorable effect of thymectomy for tumurthymia in a young myasthenic girl.
Until the middle of the 20th century, work on MG was confined to short case series.
From 1954 onwards, the application to MG with paralysis of the respiratory muscles of endotracheal artificial respiration, developed for the treatment of respiratory forms of poliomyelitis, led to the publication of large series of demyasthenics.
A report by Mollaret et al to the French Congress of Medicine in 1959 described the first successes achieved [22]. The immunological origin of MG had been presumed on the basis of a number of findings: frequency of associated autoimmune diseases; neonatal MG.
of newborns born to myasthenic mothers; frequency of myasthenic pathology; favorable action of *adrenocorticotrophic hormone* (ACTH), descorticoids, various immunosuppressants, screening for anti-organ antibodies, in particular anti-striated muscle antibodies.
The autoimmune nature of the disease put forward by Simpson in 1960[23] has since been confirmed by the production of experimental acute MG in animals, and by the presence of anti-RACh antibodies in the serum of around 85% of myasthenics.
In 1971, Engel et al used electron microscopy to describe the widening of the inter-synaptic cleft, the obliteration of folds in the post-synaptic membrane and the deposition of IgG and complement on the membrane using the immunoperoxidase technique[24].
In 1973, Fambrough et al showed a decrease in the number of RACh at the neuromuscular junction of myasthenics [25].
In 1976, Albuquerque et al observed a decrease in the sensitivity of the postsynaptic membrane to the direct application of ACh[26].
In 1976, Lindstrom developed the radioimmunoassay for anti-RACh antibodies[27].

II.2.EPIDEMIOLOGY :

MG is the most common neuromuscular junction disorder, although estimates of its frequency vary. A large number of epidemiological studies based on the MG population have been carried out worldwide since the 1950s.
A meta-analysis of 55 epidemiological studies estimated a prevalence of 77.7 per million people and an incidence of 5.3 per million people/year. However, the prevalence and incidence of MG varied markedly between the populations investigated.
Prevalence ranged from 15 to 179 per million people, and incidence from 1.7 to 21.3 cases per million people/year [28].
Consequently, in unstudied populations, prevalence and incidence rates are very difficult to extrapolate from previous studies.
Myasthenia begins at any age, from 6 months to over 80 years, and mainly affects adults under 40 (60% of cases) [29].
A study of incidence as a function of age and sex reveals a bimodal distribution, with a first peak in incidence in the 20-40 age bracket, with a *sex ratio of* 3 women to 1 man [30].
A second peak occurs in the over-50s, with a *sex ratio of* 3 men to 2 women [31].

In Korea, Health Insurance Review and Assessment (HIRA) data from 2010 to 2014 were searched for MG codes defined by ICD, 10. After identifying MG cases, we estimated annual MG prevalence and incidence based on HIRA and Korean population data. During the study period, 10138 MG cases (M: 4133, F: 6005) were identified. The prevalence of MG was 10.42 cases per 100,000 people in 2010, increasing annually to 12.99 cases per 100,000 people in 2014.

The mean incidence of MG between 2011 and 2014 was 0.69 cases per 100,000 person-years.Prevalence and incidence were higher in the older age group (≥ 50years) than in the younger age group (<50years) [prevalence: 9.26 vs. 19.24per 100,000, relative risk 2.077, 95% confidence interval 2.183, p <0.001;Incidence: 0.47 vs. 1.18 per 100,000, relative risk 2.490, 95% CI 2.006-3.091,p <0.001] [32].

II.3 Physiology of the neuromuscular junction (NMJ)

The neuron is the functional unit of the nervous system.
Each motor neuron consists of a cell body and an axon, the conducting structure of the nerve impulse. The axon divides into multiple nerve endings, located opposite the muscle fiber: the zone of communication between the nerve ending and the muscle fiber is called the neuromuscular junction (NMJ), also known as the motor plate[81].
The neuromuscular junction (NMJ), observed with a transmission electron microscope, displays the main structures characteristic of a chemical synapse:[82] it is the set of synaptic contacts between the terminal arborization of a motor axon and a striated muscle cell[83].

1) The neuromuscular synapse

The neuromuscular synapse is the junction zone between the axon of a motor neuron originating from the anterior horn of the spinal cord (presynaptic part) and the motor plate within a muscle fiber (postsynaptic part).[84]Both are separated by an intersynaptic gap or cleft of around 50 nm.[113] The neuromuscular synapse is the junction zone between the axon of a motor neuron originating from the anterior horn of the spinal cord (presynaptic part) and the motor plate within a muscle fiber (postsynaptic part).[113] Both are separated by an intersynaptic gap or cleft of around 50 nm.

***The** presynaptic zone *(the axon terminal)* is the most distal part of the motor neuron axon. It is responsible for the transformation of the electrical signal into a chemical signal.[85]At its tip, the axon undergoes an enlargement known as the terminal bouton. At the level of this knob are voltage-dependent calcium channels (Ca2+-VD channels). In addition, it contains numerous synaptic vesicles 45nm in diameter containing acetylcholine (ACh) which is the specific neurotransmitter of the motor plate; as well as a high number of mitochondria. [86]

* The synaptic cleft is the 30-50 nm thick space between the membranes of the axon terminal and the muscle cell[114].
It contains a basal lamina composed of cytoskeletal proteins, acetylcholine-degrading enzymes (*acetylcholinesterases) and* collagen[85].

*The post-synaptic membrane of the muscle fiber is embedded in shallow gutters beneath the nerve terminal, and invaginates into sub-synaptic folds about 1 to 3μm deep that open directly opposite the active zones of the presynaptic element. [114]
This so-called "junctional" membrane has a high density of nicotinic ACh receptors. (RnACh). These receptors are concentrated in the ridges of the subsynaptic folds[83].

* RnACh is a transmembrane glycoprotein resulting from the assembly of five polypeptide subunits (Pentamer): 2 alphas, 1 beta, 1 delta and 1 epsilon, delimiting a central ion channel. [115]

2) Neuromuscular transmission (TNM)

At rest, the passive release of quantas (around 10,000 ACh molecules) leads to a brief inward current known as miniature end plaque potential (MEPP), after binding and opening of the post-synaptic receptor.
The amplitude of this MEPP (0.2 to 1.2 mV) is well below the threshold required to generate a muscle action potential. [84]
During nerve stimulation, the arrival of the action potential at the presynaptic terminal leads to the opening of voltage-dependent calcium channels and thus to an increase in intracellular calcium, which in turn enables fusion between the vesicular membrane and the active zone of the nerve membrane via an important SNARE molecular complex, leading to rapid exocytosis of ACh in the synaptic cleft. [116]
Acetylcholine diffuses into the synaptic cleft and binds to its receptor. Binding of an ACh molecule to each of the two alpha subunits causes an allosteric conformational change in the receptor, resulting in opening of the ion channel and depolarization by Na entry and Na exit. [81]
This leads to a massive influx of sodium ions, producing a motor-plate potential. When this potential exceeds a critical threshold, known as the triggering threshold, voltage-dependent sodium channels (SCN4A) located at the bottom of the postsynaptic folds promote the entry of sodium ions and induce the generation of the muscle action potential and hence muscle contraction. [84]
The amplitude of the plate potential is normally much greater than that required to trigger the propagated potential, hence the term "safety margin". [81]
Any phenomenon liable to alter the interactions of ACh with its receptor will lead to a reduction in this safety margin and thus compromise TNM to a greater or lesser extent, since the amplitude of muscle cell depolarization will depend on the number of ACh-receptor interactions. If the amplitude of the plaque potential does not exceed the threshold required for depolarization, TNM fails. [117]

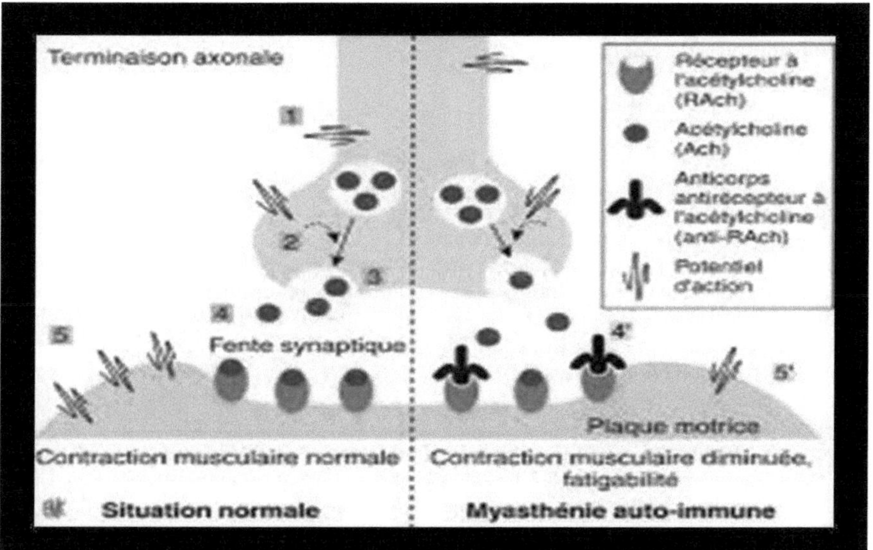

Neuromuscular junction in normal and pathological situations.
(Benchekroun, 2016)[118]

1. Arrival of an action potential at the axonal terminal
2. Gathering of acetylcholine-filled synaptic vesicles
3. Fusion of synaptic vesicles to membrane and exocytosis of neuromediator
4. Binding of acetylcholine to its receptor
5. Birth of a motor plate potential

II.4 Pathophysiology of myasthenia gravis

II.4.1 An autoimmune disease (AID)

Autoimmune diseases all result from a loss of tolerance to the self: the immune system (IS) mistakenly recognizes elements of the self and destroys them. This tolerance is normally established in the central lymphoid organs: bone marrow and thymus. The latter frequently shows abnormalities in patients with myasthenia. [87]
Myasthenia gravis is an acquired autoimmune disorder caused by impaired neuromuscular transmission due to post-synaptic neuromuscular blockade of motor-plate receptors by anti-acetylcholine receptor antibodies (Ac anti-RAch). **88.**So the origin of this disease is thought to be linked to T lymphocytes (LT),
which control the B lymphocytes (LB) that manufacture antibodies. **[89]**

1- Autoantibodies :
Depending on the series and detection methods used, anti-RACh, anti-MuSK and anti-LRP4 antibodies are found in 70-80%, 1-10% and 1-33% of patients respectively. Other antibodies are known, but their pathogenicity remains debated. [**90**]

1-1- Anti-acetylcholine receptor antibodies:

The acetylcholine receptor is composed of five subunits. Anti-RACh antibodies are most often directed against an extracellular epitope of the two alpha subunits. Antibodies directed against the beta subunit appear to be less pathogenic. [**91**]
Anti-RACh is predominantly of the IgG1 and IgG3 classes, and therefore has the ability to activate the classical complement pathway**.** Light chain isotypes are of the Kappa subtype. They possess polyclonal activity directed against all RACh subunits, with preferential tropism for an α-subunit binding site different from the ACh-binding region known as the *main immunogenicregion (MIR)*. [92]
The presence of these antibodies is found in 80-90% of patients with generalized myasthenia and only in 50% of subjects with pure ocular myasthenia. [**93]**
The anti-RACh titre does not correlate with the severity of myasthenia. Nevertheless, a parallelism between anti-RACh titer and disease progression has been reported: an increase in titer seems predictive of a relapse, whereas a stable or decreasing level is observed in stabilized forms**. [94]**
In 16% to 38% of seronegative patients using conventional techniques (immunoprecipitation), low-affinity anti-RACh antibodies can be detected using more sensitive methods (cell transfection). These antibodies recognize aggregated RACh. [95]

* Pathogenicity of anti-RACh antibodies: [100].

Anti-acetylcholine receptor antibodies are pathogenic, and proceed via 4 distinct mechanisms which lead to a decrease in the level of functional receptors. As a result, nerve conduction to the muscle fiber is remarkably impaired.

- The main mechanism is the destruction of the postsynaptic membrane under the influence of complement C5b-B9 (membrane attack complex).
- Antigenic modulation also occurs, corresponding to accelerated internalization of RACh with endocytosis and intracellular proteolytic degradation by lysosomal enzymes.

▪ There is also a direct blockade of the ACh binding site at the post-synaptic membrane, known as the *curare-like* effect, which is the least significant.

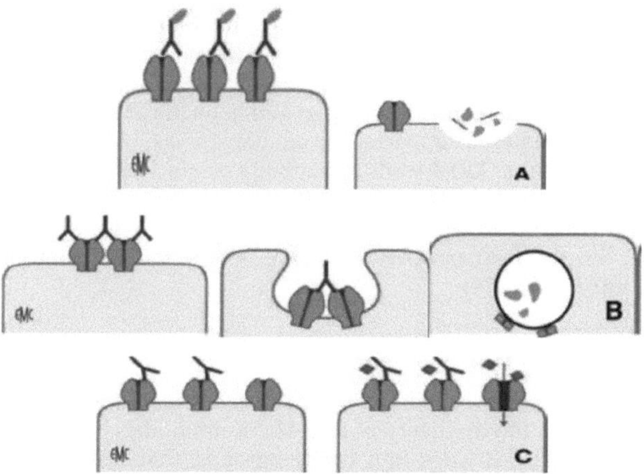

Figure 5: Mechanism of action of anti-acetylcholine receptor antibodies
(Bensafi et al., 2015)[96]

A. Complement-induced destruction of the postsynaptic membrane
B. Degradation of membrane receptors by endocytosis
C. Antibody blocking action

1-2- Kinase-specific anti-muscle autoantibodies

In 40% of generalized myasthenias without anti-RACh, antibodies are detected against another post-synaptic molecule, MuSK (Muscle specefic Kinase), which is a tyrosine-phospho-kinase involved in RACh transcription and its membrane anchoring.

Unlike patients with anti-RACh antibodies, there is a good correlation between anti-MuSK antibody levels and clinical severity in this category of patients. [97]

MuSK (Muscle specific Kinase) is a post-synaptic transmembrane protein described in1995 that is involved in a signaling pathway integrating agrin, LRP4, rapsyne anddownstream of tyrosine kinase 7 (DOK7) and leading to RACh aggregation.[98] It is also involved in RACh aggregation.

Anti-MuSKs are of the IgG4 class and therefore cannot activate complement. However, their direct pathogenicity has been demonstrated by passive transfer studies in animals and appears to be linked to blockage of MuSK- LRP4 binding, resulting in a defect in RACh aggregation. [99]

Anti-MuSK antibodies also inhibit the proliferation of myoblasts in vitro and satellite cells in vivo. Taken together, these data show that anti-MuSK antibodies have a clear pathogenic effect both in vitro and in vivo, and that their mode of action is clearly different from anti-RACh antibodies. [100]

1-3- Anti-LRP4 antibodies

LRP4 is a post-synaptic protein in the agrin-LRP4-MuSK signaling pathway. LRP4 and MuSK are pre-assembled, but MuSK activation is induced by agrin binding to LRP4 **(Koneczny and Herbst, 2019).**

Anti-LRP4 antibodies block agrin-LRP4 interaction, leading to inhibition of post-synaptic RACh clustering and disruption of MuSK activation. 102] They are mainly igG1- and igG2-class antibodies and can therefore activate complementation. 103] They also interfere with agrin binding to its receptor and modify RACh aggregation on muscle cells. [104]

The pathogenicity of these antibodies is supported by animal studies: immunization of mice with the extracellular domain of LRP4 leads to antibody production and the onset of myasthenic symptoms, and passive transfer of anti-LRP4 to naïve mice results in signs of myasthenia. [90]

Anti-LRP4 is detected in 1-5% of myasthenic patients and in 7-33 of double-seronegative patients (anti-RACh and anti-Musk). [94]

2- Seronegative myasthenia :

Historically, the term "seronegative myasthenia" referred to myasthenias not associated with anti-RACh antibodies. Since the discovery of anti-MuSK antibodies, this group of seronegative myasthenias has been divided into two subgroups, that associated with anti-MuSK and a so-called "double seronegative" group without anti-RACh and without anti-MuSK. The latter are very similar in distribution, course and response to treatment to the forms associated with anti-RACh antibodies. [116]

In fact, low-affinity anti-RACh antibodies are found in 66% of these so-called seronegative forms.

These antibodies, undetectable by standard immunoprecipitation techniques, have been demonstrated on cell preparations expressing clostered RACh[90].

3-Myasthenia and thymus :

The thymus is a lymphoid organ located in the lower part of the neck, behind the breastbone, in front of the trachea and at the top of the thorax. It is the origin of T-lymphocyte maturation.

It plays a fundamental role in the induction of tolerance to self, allowing intrathymic destruction of autoreactive effector T cells (negative selection) and maturation of regulatory T cells. [84]

In addition, abnormalities in the thymic selection of RACh-specific effector and regulatory T cells have been described in myasthenia gravis. [109]

Under physiological conditions, the majority cell types in the thymus are thymocytes and stromal cells.

In the majority of myasthenic patients, the thymus shows structural and functional changes characterized by the presence of germinal centers containing a large number of B cells, which is defined as follicular hyperplasia, or by the presence of a tumor (thymoma). [100]

a) Follicular hyperplasia :

Expression of the RACh autoantigen by thymic epithelial cells and myoid cells (non-mature muscle cells expressing RAChfoetal and adult) contributes to the selection of specific T lymphocytes driving the inflammatory response and production of anti-RACh antibodies in germinal center follicles. Functional abnormalities of regulatory T cells involved in apoptosis of autoreactive T lymphocytes have also been described. [119]

b) Thymoma :

activation of B lymphocytes in the extrathymic immune system by autoreactive T effector cells after their intratumoral thymic maturation [90].

In addition, tumor architectural disorganization, selective loss of regulatory T cells and abnormalities in the expression of genes that regulate the immune response, such as the AIRE (Auto-immune Regulator) gene, a key factor in immune tolerance, favor the generation of autoreactive T lymphocytes. [112]

III.DIAGNOSIS OF MYASTHENIA :

III.1.POSITIVE DIAGNOSIS :

The general practitioner is often the first professional contacted by the patient at the start of his myasthenia. The diagnosis should be made in the presence of the following symptoms and clinical signs, which should be investigated by questioning, clinical examination [29] and paraclinical tests.

III.1.1 Examination :

III.1.1.1The motor deficit :

It is the main symptom [29] in 1 in 5 patients [106]. It is highly variable and unsystematized, affecting only one muscle, or one or more muscle groups (upper or lower limbs) with voluntary control of the body, without correlation with a nerve root or trunk.

The essential fact is the myasthenic phenomenon:

- Fatigue on exertion: the deficit is generally proportional to the intensity and duration of exertion, always more intense at the end of the day, aggravated by cold, emotions and digestion, improved by rest (progressive recovery).

The deficit does not always occur in the muscle group in question [20].

III.1.1.2 Trunk and limb involvement :

Fatigue of the shoulder girdle, so patients may complain of difficulty in lifting their arms, climbing stairs or simply walking, and in performing everyday tasks such as styling their hair, washing their hair, opening a bottle or even writing[37].

A deficit in the neck extensor muscles, with the head falling forward (frequent in severe forms) [42]; this is the only weakness that can generate pain, in the form of posterior cervical myalgia, linked to a phenomenon of relaxation [37, 38]; damage to the finger extensors is particularly frequent.

In the lower limbs, unexplained falls may reveal myasthenia gravis, particularly when exercising.

Limb involvement mainly affects the limb girdles.

Axial involvement (trunk and abdominal muscles) predominates over cervical muscles.

Facial muscle damage can result in facial diplegia (facial paralysis). It is often minimal, with an inexpressive appearance of the face, accentuated during lamimicus, and the impossibility of inflating the cheeks or whistling [42].

III.1.1.3 Oculopalpebral muscle involvement :

This condition is the most common, but also the most suggestive, as it is often overlooked in the medical field [19].

Involvement of the eye muscles is virtually constant, and is often the only manifestation in the early stages.

- Uni- or bilateral ptosis, usually asymmetrical [42], corresponding to drooping eyelids. It worsens at the end of the day and when the patient is asked to "open his eyes". In addition to fatigue, it may be accentuated by light or provoked by forced elevation of the globesocularis.

Intrinsic motility is respected [19]. It is frequently accompanied by compensatory contraction of the frontal muscle [42].

A ptosis may appear when walking or chewing.

- The extra-ocular muscle involved in eye movement is also affected (oculomotor damage). It causes diplegia (double vision) [114], the most frequent symptom, isolated or associated with ptosis. It may be horizontal or oblique. It often appears in the late evening [42].

Patients often complain of difficulty reading, driving, watching television, etc.

Typically, fatigue, bright lights and fixation on an object will accentuate these two signs [37].

The vegetative pupillary musculature is never affected (normal light-motor reflex).

Some forms of myasthenia are confined to the oculomotor muscles (pure oculomotor myasthenia), while more diffuse forms are referred to as generalized myasthenia.

III.1.1.4 Bulbar involvement :

the involvement of bulbar innervation muscles can be the cause of dysphonia with phonation disorders (nasal voice), frequently triggered by emotions [42], swallowing disorders due to deficits in the masticatory muscles [19] should be investigated with particular care, as they can be life-threatening: dysphagia favored by hot food, sometimes with false routes [42], and difficulties in mastication should also prompt a diagnosis.

If these signs are present, the patient must be transferred to intensive care.

III.1.1.5 Respiratory disease :

The seriousness of this autoimmune disease lies in its potential to affect respiratory muscles, which can be life-threatening and requires emergency treatment.

In more moderate cases, this can lead to dyspnea on exertion, or even at rest [38].

III.1.2 Diagnosis of severity :

It is essential to identify signs of severity. The onset of respiratory problems within a few days, with congestion, shortness of breath, ineffective coughing, false coughs and rapid motor deterioration, should lead to the diagnosis of a **crisis.**

life-threatening **myasthenia.**

It is an absolute emergency, requiring immediate admission to intensive care in order to initiate ventilatory assistance if necessary, and to secure food supply (gastric tube). Involvement of the respiratory and trunk muscles, which can occur in severe forms, is rarely an initial symptom, and may be caused by respiratory infection or inappropriate use of curariforms [42].

Listening to the patient is essential: the repetition of symptoms, their coherence and originality (nasal voice, misdirection, diplopia) should challenge the practitioner, who must not trivialize them.
A new consultation should be organized as soon as symptoms appear, especially at the end of the day. Once the hypothesis has been raised, the general practitioner must refer the patient as quickly as possible to a specialist able to confirm the diagnosis (neurologist, neuropediatrician). Delaying exposes the patient to a severe relapse, which can occur within a few days [29].

III.1.3 Clinical examination
The diagnosis of myasthenia gravis is essentially clinical:

- reduced muscle strength when certain movements are repeated
- Apart from thrusts, muscle strength is initially normal and only decreases with repetition of movements [20].

A specific chronology with symptom variability, either stereotyped and predictable (increase in the evening or at the time of menstruation), or part of an unexpected flare-up, corresponding to a worsening of the disease over a period of several weeks to several months.
The ptosis is particularly instructive, as it can vary within minutes and/or alternate, thus demonstrating variability and providing an unmistakable sign of myasthenic syndrome. Photographic images are useful for assessing variability: if there is significant ptosis [29].
The myasthenic origin of a ptosis can also be evoked by the positivity of the ice cube test: with the patient's eyelids closed, an ice cube is applied (via a compress) to one side of the eyelid for 3 to 4 minutes; when the ice cube is removed, the ptosis disappears on that side, and sometimes even on the other. The improvement is short-lived but certain.

- negative signs: rest of examination normal: osteotendinous reflexes are normal. There are no sensory or sphincter disturbances. Muscular atrophy is exceptional, but may be observed in myasthenias.
- look for other signs of autoimmune disease (dysthyroidism, vitiligo, anemia, lupus, polyarthritis).

The neurological examination is often strictly normal at rest, and it is exertion that brings on the symptoms [20].

III.1.3.1 Clinical assessment
Myasthenia is assessed by scores, and among the most widely used are the motor score (the Garches score) and the daily activity score (over the last 8 days). (See Appendix 1), which also enable objective assessment of treatment.

III.1.4 Additional tests :

The purpose of these examinations is to confirm the diagnosis, inform and educate the patient, assess severity, look for associated disease (thymoma, autoimmune disease), establish therapeutic indications and, if possible, refer to a specialist consultation [29].

III.1.4.1 An electromyogram (EMG)
It is particularly useful in seronegative forms and when rapid diagnosis is required. Repetitive stimulation tests at 2 or 3 Hz aim to reduce the amplitude of muscular evoked

responses, in principle by more than 10%. If possible, they should be performed first on the territories clinically concerned. Their sensitivity varies from 25% for thecubital to almost 90% for the circumflex in generalized myasthenia; it is less than 50% in pure ocular myasthenia [43]. Care must be taken to ensure that the muscles studied are sufficiently warm, as low temperatures can result in false negatives.
Anticholinesterase drugs should also be avoided if possible [42] the day before the examination [29].
Single-fiber EMG has better sensitivity [42,29] (over 80% for pure ocular forms and 95% for generalized forms) [42], revealing jitter prolongation (time interval between the potentials of two muscle fibers of the same motor unit), which is delicate and time-consuming to perform, and should be reserved for difficult cases (negativity of classic ENMG, particularly in ocular myasthenia or in certain cases of myasthenia with anti-MuSK ouseronegative antibodies).
In children, classical single-fiber studies are not possible due to lack of cooperation, and repetitive stimulation studies can be difficult. Stimulated single-fiber studies are possible (without the need for cooperation) in some specialized centers. This study is more sensitive but less specific for the diagnosis of neuromuscular junction disorders than the repetitive stimulation study [29].
It should be emphasized that these tests have no specificity. They simply measure the safety margin of the JNM.
Clinical examination and conventional ENMG techniques must verify the absence of other pathologies to allow correct interpretation of the results [42].
When a motor nerve is repeatedly stimulated in a deficit area, there is an amplitude decrement (progressive, transient decrease) in motor unit potentials, whereas a single stimulation is normal. The decrease in response is followed by a plateau phase or an increase [20]. A decrement is significant if the decrease in amplitude is greater than 10% auminimum over 2 muscle pairs, during repetitive stimulation at 3 cycles/second in electroneuromyography. It must be sought on several muscle nerve pairs, proximal and distal, as well as the cephalic extremity [29].

III.1.4.2 Testing for anti-acetylcholine receptor antibodies (anti-AChR)
This is the most specific test. The presence of antibodies establishes the diagnosis [42]. Antibodies are detected by radioimmunoassay or enzyme assay [Elisa], with results that are essentially equivalent.
These are polyclonal antibodies of the IgG class, detected in around 85% of myasthenic patients [42,44], with no close parallel between their levels and the clinical state from one patient to another [20,44]; their titre is most often low in ocular forms, where they are found in only 50% of cases [42,45], and high in generalized forms, especially when there is thymic hyperplasia or thymoma [45]. Their reduction generally goes hand in hand with clinical improvement, rapid after plasma exchange (PE), slow after thymic hyperplasia.
after thymectomy, corticoids, immunosuppressants.
Anti-RACh antibody assays are primarily of diagnostic value, but repeated assays are useful for assessing the effects of different treatments. A rise in antibody levels may accompany, or even precede, clinical relapse[46,47].
The responsibility of anti-RACh antibodies in the onset of MG is attested by autoimmune myasthenia, by the rapid improvement in motor deficit after PE, by neonatal MG, and by the deposition of IgG and complement on the post-synaptic membrane, whose folds are erased.

They can act via three mechanisms to cause the loss of functional RACh [48]:
- complement-dependent lysis of the post-synaptic membrane ;
- accelerated degradation of RACh by endocytosis ;
- blocking ACh binding sites.
specificity is not perfect. False positives may be encountered in other autoimmune conditions, in particular Lambert-Eaton myasthenic syndrome, hyperthyroidism, amyotrophic lateral sclerosis, during treatment with D-penicillamine and in parents of myasthenics [42].

III.1.4.3 Anti-MuSK (muscle-specific kinase) antibody test
Known long before anti-RACh antibodies, anti-striated muscle antibodies were first detected by immunofluorescence and then by other immunological techniques (immunoprecipitation technique) [29].

III.1.4.4 Chest X-ray and thymic CT scan
Injection-free thoracic CT scans [29] to investigate thymic abnormalities, whether thymomas or simple thymic remnants with varying degrees of hyperplasia (present in around 20% of myasthenia gravis cases), should always be performed as a matter of course. If there is any doubt about a thymoma, particularly in young adults with a dense thymus, an iodine injection may be indicated, but this may aggravate unstable myasthenia [29].

III.1.4.5 EFR (respiratory function tests)
In generalized forms, look for respiratory involvement [49].

III.1.5 Therapeutic and diagnostic testing
The clinical examination is completed by a therapeutic test: IV or IM injection.
an ampoule of prostigmine or edrophonium. A pharmacological test with edrophonium (tensilon) one ampoule (10mg), slowly injecting 2mg of the product in a strict IV to detect any hypersensitivity of the patient to muscarinic effects; if all goes well, the remaining 8mg are injected in an IV over 30 seconds to 1 minute.The patient is monitored for improvement. The duration of action is 2 to 20 minutes, but can reach 2 hours in patients on corticosteroids.
Respiratory function must be carefully assessed before the
so that the patient can be rapidly intubated if tensilon induces apnea[20] or prostigmine (reversol) (short-acting anticholinesterase agents), whose action takes longer to appear (1 to 2 hours) and disappears in 3 or 4 hours. The usual dose is 0.4mg/Kg IM [20].
This test confirms the diagnosis by making clinical signs transiently disappear or improve within a maximum of 15 minutes [49].
It is useful when the improvement of a deficit can be easily quantified: ptosis, diplopia, voice weakness, swallowing disorder.
Muscarinic effects can be avoided by injecting 0.4mg of atropine as a preventive measure or when they appear.

NOTE: Negative results do not rule out the diagnosis [29,49], since neither the tensilon/Reversol test, nor the presence of EMG decrement, nor the presence of anti-AChR is 100% sensitive [49].

If symptoms persist or worsen [29], or if a new symptom appears [29,49], the patient must be seen again. Repeat the specific antibody assay a few months after the 1st assay, as secondary specific antibody positivity is possible, especially if myasthenia gravis has worsened. If diplopia or eyelid droop is isolated, and especially if it does not fluctuate, a cerebral MRI is recommended to rule out a cerebral, tumoral or vascular lesion [29].

III.2 Classification: Types of myasthenia gravis

The MGFA and Osserman classifications are used to assess extension of symptoms and severity of disease, also MGFA status post which allows the patient's condition to be monitored after the procedure (see appendix 02).

III.3 Disease progression

The most frequent initial clinical presentation of this pathology is a ocular weakness [38] with ptosis and diplopia, but after one year of evolution in 80-90% of patients, other territories are affected [29].

In 17% of patients, the disease remains localized to the ocular muscles after 2 years, in which case we can speak of pure ocular myasthenia gravis [38] .

This form is more common in men over the age of 40 [29].

It is estimated that 13% of patients will have bulbar symptoms associated with their ocular weakness; for 20%, it will be associated with limb fatigability; and finally, for 50% of myasthenia patients, the weakness will be generalized to many, or even almost all, voluntary muscles. This is known as generalized myasthenia gravis.

Spontaneous remissions are rare; according to the latest estimates, they may nevertheless occur in 10-20% of patients. They occur mainly in cases of iatrogenic autoimmune myasthenia gravis, and are generally reversible on discontinuation [38].

Worsening phases are usually characterized by the onset of successive flare-ups, sometimes triggered by physical or psychological stress, and sometimes following remissions and a tendency to worsen in the first few years. These flare-ups vary in severity, and sometimes require hospitalization to balance treatment: for 85% of patients, the maximum severity of the disease is reached in less than 3 years.

The severity of myasthenia must be assessed at each consultation, on the basis of both examination and questioning. The severity of myasthenia gravis varies greatly from patient to patient and, within the same patient, from one moment to the next [29].

III.3.1 Myasthenic attacks

Weakness may decompensate more or less rapidly during the worsening phases, which may occur more or less frequently depending on the case. These are characterized by a worsening of symptoms, which can go as far as to include respiratory muscle damage and severe swallowing disorders [37], which characterize severe forms of the disease (20-30% of patients) [29], where intensive care with assisted ventilation and/or intubation has considerably reduced mortality.

Patients and their GPs will need to learn to recognize the warning signs [29,50] that may indicate a new, severe attack, in order to limit their progression as quickly as possible [50], and thus require an emergency consultation [29]. These symptoms include, of course, a recurrence or worsening of symptoms present before treatment, and a high level of generalized fatigue: fatigability during light exertion, voice changes or speech difficulties, swallowing difficulties [29,50], the emergency is absolute and requires urgent

hospitalization in intensive care, in the event of rapid progression of symptoms, the onset of breathlessness, coughing difficulties, false routes compromising feeding, all signs heralding a myasthenic crisis [29].
These flare-ups can be caused by a variety of factors, including environmental, physical, psychological and medication-related.
Aggravating factors include infection, intense exercise of course, shock or emotional stress, elevated body temperature, menstruation for some women, pregnancy, surgery [37,50], as well as drugs that interfere with the functioning of the JNM or with the treatment of myasthenia gravis, as we shall see later [38].
Thanks to immunotherapeutic advances, these attacks are becoming less frequent in patients under our care.
However, depending on the source, they range from less than 2% of patients [50] to around 20-30% [51,52].
In contrast, myasthenia remains mild in 25% of patients.
Between these two extremes, the disease is of intermediate severity, incapacitating due to marked fatigability, swallowing and chewing disorders, a nasal voice, and marked oculomotor impairment (diplopia and/or ptosis) [29].

Circumstances justifying hospitalization in intensive care :

- swallowing disorders, false route.
- breathing difficulties, dyspnea, all ineffective.
- rapidly extensive muscle strength deficit.
- resistance to well-administered anticholinesterase therapy [29].

III.4 Follow-up :

Follow-up of this condition, whose evolution is capricious with a risk of abrupt worsening, is ensured jointly by the specialist in charge of the patient and the attending physician, who is in the front line to monitor treatment, detect worsening of the myasthenia and any complications due to the toxicity of cortisone or immunosuppressive treatment.
Myasthenia gravis falls within the scope of long-term illnesses, which are reimbursed at 100%.
The attending physician will assist the patient in becoming a "player" in his or her pathology, by providing comprehensive information on the course of the disease, aggravating factors, prognosis, the different treatments, their side-effects, how to take them (particularly anticholinesterase drugs), how to recognize signs of seriousness and what to do in the event of them (rapid consultation, recourse to hospital emergency services, or even mobile emergency services).
The myasthenia card is an essential tool to be given to the patient at the first consultation. Drug contraindications are clearly listed, to guide the attending physician in any prescription [29].

III.5 Myasthenia and associated pathologies :

III.5.1. Myasthenia and autoimmune diseases :

The association of myasthenia with another autoimmune disease is not exceptional, conditions are varied. In the same patient, several autoimmune diseases may be associated with myasthenia gravis, each evolving independently [29]In his series of 784 patients, Oosterhuis counted 10% of autoimmune diseases associated with myasthenia gravis in men and 26% in women [106].

In addition, autoimmune disorders are often found in close relatives.

Dysthyroidism is the most frequently associated condition (5-10% of patients) [29]. They predominate in all major literature series. Various autoimmune inflammatory pathologies may accompany myasthenia gravis: rheumatoid arthritis (the second most common condition: 2% [53] to 4% [106]), Gougerot-Sjogren's, Systemic Lupus Erythematosus (SLE: 1% [53] to 1.5% [106]).

Myositis may be associated with myasthenia with or without thymoma. Both conditions induce muscle weakness, which can complicate diagnosis.

Elevated CPK levels, absent in myasthenia, point to inflammatory myopathy confirmed by muscle biopsy, which often reveals a granulomatous myositis form, frequently associated with a thymoma.

The prognosis for these myositis-myasthenia associations is often severe, with the risk of death from cardiac and/or respiratory complications.

III.5.2 Myasthenia and neuromuscular disorders :

Other neuromuscular disorders associated with myasthenia have been described: Lambert-Eaton syndrome, neuromuscular hyperexcitability syndrome (neuromyotonia) due to antibodies directed against potassium channels in motor nerve endings; arguments in favor of diagnosis are the presence of myokimia, to be distinguished from simple fasciculations caused by anticholinesterase drugs, neuropathic pain, possibly hypersudation and sleep or memory disturbances, the appearance of motor unit potentials, doublets, triplets or multiplets on ENMG, and the presence of antibodies directed against potassium channels in the motor nerve (anti-CASPR2), detected in more than half of cases.In cases of myasthenia/neuromyotonia, a thymoma is frequently associated.

III.6 Clinical forms of myasthenia gravis

III.6.1. Ocular myasthenia :

In 50% of cases, MG begins with ocular signs. Among cases of MG

Initially limited to the eye, half of all myasthenias later remain localized there; extension to other territories occurs in the majority of cases within 2 years of onset, and is more frequent after the age of 50 [54]. Although ocular myasthenia is considered benign due to its localized nature, it can be very troublesome due to the extent of diplopia. The characteristics of ocular myasthenia in adults are as follows:

- predominantly male,
- age of onset usually over 40,
- rarity of thymoma.
- Frank variability, of which alternating ptosis is the most characteristic manifestation, is very useful in making the diagnosis, which is above all clinical, since anti-RACh antibodies are absent in half of all cases, the response to anticholinesterase

drugs is frequently absent or weak, and conventional electroneuromyography is frequently negative, including at orbicular level. Single-fiber study of the facial territory has a much higher diagnostic yield[29].

–

III.6.2 Myasthenia associated with anti-MuSK antibodies :

Approximately 15% of patients have no anti-RACh antibodies although they have characteristic clinical signs of MG.
Nevertheless, there is strong evidence that their disease is mediated by autoantibodies [55].
MuSK is involved in RACh clustering during synapse formation, but is also expressed in the mature neuromuscular junction. Anti-MuSK antibodies inhibit MuSK function in cultured myotubes with high affinity.
There are therefore two immunologically distinct forms of MG.
In addition, seronegative myasthenic patients usually have normal thymuses [56]. Testing for anti-MuSK antibodies, which is possible with a simple Elisa test, is very useful for diagnosing seronegative forms in adults and children, and also helps to exclude thymoma, particularly in patients with anti-RACh antibodies.
The characteristics of myasthenia with anti-MuSK antibodies are as follows:

- a strong preponderance of women at all ages,
- generalized nature of myasthenia,
- marked severity with significant bulbar and respiratory involvement, requiring immunosuppressive treatment,
- presence of lingual and masseterine atrophy,
- thymic involution,
- absence of thymoma.
- The disappointing response to anticholinesterase drugs,
- the frequent negativity of electroneuromyographic exploration (absence of decrement) complicates the diagnosis [36].

III.6.3. Myasthenia associated with low-affinity anti-RACh and anti-LRP4 :
Lrp4 has been identified as a post-synaptic protein crucial for the development and maintenance of the neuromuscular junction [57] with function
as the agrin receptor required for MuSK activation[58, 59].
Anti-Lrp4 has been hypothesized to be a pathogenic factor in seronegative MG due to its postsynaptic localization and observations in Lrp4-deficient animal models showing a phenotype similar to that observed in MuSK-negative animals [60,61]. [Capable of activating complement and thus producing damage to the postsynaptic lamina via the membrane attack complex.
In addition, inhibition of agrin-induced aggregation of RACh in the muscle-end plate has been implicated as a pathogenic mechanism in Lrp4-MG.
Myasthenias associated with low-affinity anti-RACh and anti-LRP4 antibodies are similar to those of classical anti-RACh myasthenia:

- female dominance
- involvement in generalized (usually mild if anti-LRP4 antibodies) and ocular forms,
- involutive or hyperplastic thymus [29].

III.6.4 Myasthenia gravis and pregnancy :

Fertility is not affected by the disease, so pregnancy is not uncommon in myasthenia gravis.
During pregnancy, there is a serious risk of exacerbation of myasthenic symptoms in 30 to 40% of cases [20,29,49], especially in the first three months and even more so in the days and first weeks after delivery (postpartum) [29,49], which is why reinforced monitoring is necessary: risk of relapse [49].
It is therefore advisable to give birth in a facility where mother and child can be cared for in intensive care [29], but the condition may also be stationary (1/3), or improve (1/3) [20,49].

- therapeutic abortion is not indicated, as it may aggravate the disease.
- during labor, anticholinesterase agents are used parenterally.
- local or regional anaesthesia is preferable to general anaesthesia, and care must be taken when using sedatives.
- Caesarean sections are only performed when indicated by the obstetrician.
- the neurologist and obstetrician must help myasthenic women to

plan their pregnancies. Voluntary sterilization or contraception should be suggested when myasthenia gravis is severe [20].

IV. DIFFERENTIAL DIAGNOSIS :

IV.1 Lambert-Eaton syndrome (LES) :

Myasthenic (or myastheniform) syndrome caused by the presence of antibodies voltage-dependent anti-synaptic calcium channels; these antibodies prevent the release of acetylcholine at the synaptic terminal:

- Paraneoplastic in 75% of cases (look for anaplastic small-cell lung cancer as a priority). Most often, SMEL precedes the discovery of cancer.

-In favour of a paraneoplastic origin, the following will be considered

- terrain (men over 40, smokers),
- association with other paraneoplastic manifestations (cerebellar syndrome, neuropathy, especially if painful and/or ataxic),
- the presence of anti-SOX antibodies.

The absence of anti-calcium channel antibodies favors a non-calcium channel form of the disease.
paraneoplastic[29].

- associated with an autoimmune disease (lupus, dysthyroidism, Biermer's anemia, Gougerot-Sjogren's) in 10% of cases. An association with HLA haplotypes B8 and DR3 has been reported [42].
- Idiopathic in 10% of cases.

The most frequent symptom is fatigability (proximal deficit) of the lower limbs, with discrete oculobulbar signs often limited to mild ptosis, but the motor deficit improves with repeated effort, through recruitment of calcium channels - unlike in myasthenia where the motor deficit worsens with effort [29].

IV.2.Drug-induced or toxic myasthenic syndromes (iatrogenic myasthenic syndromes) :

Myasthenic syndrome is secondary to the use of substances likely to

The rapid improvement on discontinuation of treatment supports the involvement of the treatment.
Certain toxic substances, such as manganese and snake venoms containing neurotoxins, can interfere with the functioning of the neuromuscular junction, resulting in acute and severe myastheniform syndromes (acetylcholine receptor blockade). Diagnosis by anamnesis is often straightforward [29].

IV.3. Botulism :
Botulism is a rare but serious cause of presynaptic myasthenic syndrome[29]. It is an infectious disease linked to the action of the toxin of clostridium botulinum, which is contracted by ingesting spoiled home-made canned food. The bacterium produces a toxin that inhibits voltage-dependent calcium channels, resulting in reduced release of acetylcholine into the synaptic cleft:
-onset of symptoms 12 to 24 hours after ingestion of tainted canned food, but also after heroin injection
- digestive problems (nausea, vomiting)
- dry mouth [29]
- diplopia ptosis and mydriasis,
- disorders of phonation, swallowing and breathing.
- a progressively generalized downward motor deficit, associated with urinary retention, constipation, lacrimal and salivary hyposecretion.
Diagnosis is confirmed by identification of botulinum toxin in blood and/or food.

V.THERAPEUTIC MANAGEMENT :

V.1.Principle :

Every case of autoimmune myasthenia is different, and will therefore require individualized management, depending on the patient's clinical presentation, the impact of the disease on daily life, the subtype of myasthenia (age of onset, type of antibodies, presence or absence of a thymoma), comorbidities, patient compliance...[36].

V.2.Objectives :

Treatment has several objectives: to reduce symptoms and their impact on personal and professional life as much as possible, to manage serious complications threatening vital functions, and to limit the progression of the disease. In addition to the severity of the motor deficit, it must take into account treatment tolerance, therapeutic risks (by minimizing adverse drug reactions), the social and professional impact of the disease, and the patient's expectations [29]. It is a chronic disease, for which there is currently no cure: Treatment can stabilize myasthenia gravis and, in some cases, even bring about remission [39].
Although currently available treatments have dramatically reduced mortality, autoimmune myasthenia gravis remains a rare disease, and few large-scale, placebo-controlled clinical trials over a sufficiently long time scale are available [37]. Current recommendations are essentially based on experience and clinical consensus [51].

V.3 Available treatments and their uses :

There are essentially two types of treatment, which may be combined: the However, no treatment is specific to myasthenia gravis, and most of the treatments discussed here were initially prescribed for other, mainly autoimmune, diseases [36].

V.3.1 Symptomatic treatment (anticholinesterase drugs) :

V.3.1.1 Anticholinesterase agents :

It is based on anticholinesterase agents, which oppose acetylcholine degradation in the synaptic cleft (prolonging the action of acetylcholine at the post-synaptic membrane by reversible blockade of acetylcholineesterase) [49], thus offsetting the effect of anti-RACh autoantibodies.

This is the cornerstone of therapeutic management of autoimmune myasthenia gravis, the first-line treatment [38].

In milder forms of myasthenia gravis, this treatment is often sufficient[49].

This treatment is not very effective in people with autoimmune myasthenia with anti-MuSK[63].

Pyridostigmine bromide (Mestinon®), ambemonium chloride (Mytelase®) and neostigmine (Prostigmine°) are the only drugs approved for use in myasthenia gravis.

They constitute the basic symptomatic treatment of myasthenia and are the first treatment to be initiated in cases of suspected or confirmed myasthenia [29].

They differ from each other in terms of their onset and duration of action, and in their muscarinic effects, which are more marked for Prostigmine and Mytelase than for Mestinon; Mytelase has the longest effect.

Mestinon and Mytelase have an almost similar pharmacokinetic profile, with an onset of action around 30 minutes after ingestion and a duration of action of around 4 hours [64]. They will therefore provide only a temporary improvement in muscle strength [37].

Mestinon® LP or Mestinon retard® (180 mg) is also available in extended-release pyridostigmine form, and requires an ATU (Autorisation Temporaired'Utilisation) in hospital pharmacies [65]. With a duration of action of 6 to 8 hours, this presentation is useful for maintaining an effective level of anticholinesterase during the night, and thus avoiding swallowing disorders on awakening (morning dysphagia) in certain patients, who take the drug at bedtime [29].

Like all quaternary ammonium compounds, these drugs are poorly resorbed in the intestine, partly through the formation of non-resorbable complexes with mucin and bile salts.

The combined intake of food significantly reduces their absorption [66].and so they do not pass the Hemato-Encephalic Barrier [67].

Treatment is adapted by successive adjustments, often starting with an average dose of 60 mg pyridostigmine (mestinon°) every 4 hours, or an equivalent treatment.

Parenteral treatments are used in the event of an acute attack, after surgery, or if dysphagia is a cause for concern. The parenteral dose is one-thirtieth of the oral dose for neostigmine or pyridostigmine.

Side effects are reduced if the drugs are taken with meals and in divided doses. Atropine may be combined with ginatropin° (0.4 to 0.8 mg po) at the start of treatment.

Dénomination	Posologie et durée d'action
La néostigmine (prostigmine°)	Cp sécables à 15 mg : 5 à 20 cp/j en 4 à 6 prises. Durée d'action 2 h.
La pyridostigmine (mestinon°) Délai d'action= 30min Durée d'action= 3 à 4h	Cp à 60 mg : 4 à 8 cp/j en 3 à 4 prises. Durée d'action 4 h.
L'ambenomium (mytelase°) Délai d'action= 30 min Durée d'action= 4 à 6 h	Cp sécables à 10 mg : 3 à 10cp/j en 3 à 4 prises. Durée d'action 5 à 6 h.
La néostigmine (prostigmine°) Délai d'action=10 à 15 min Durée d'action= 1 à 2h	Ampoule à 0.5 mg : 2 à 5 amp/jr en 4 à 6 injections par voie SC ou IM
L'edrophonium (tensilon°)	Ampoule à 10mg IV strict

V.3.1.2 Rules for use :

A number of rules must be observed when prescribing them:
-Taken on an empty stomach 30 min to 1 h before meals [49], their action starts on average 30 m after ingestion and lasts around 4 h.
A 4-hour interval should preferably be observed between two doses [29].
-Intakes should be spread out over the day, depending on how the patient's symptoms evolve over the course of the day, and on the patient's activities and lifestyle. For example, a patient with swallowing difficulties should take the anticholinesterase 30 minutes before each meal, to limit the risk of false swallowing.
-Therapeutic education is important here, as patients need to know how to regulate their intake without exceeding the tolerance threshold, which could then accentuate muscular disorders[39]. To achieve this, patients need to be fully informed of the treatment's mode of action and pharmacokinetic characteristics.
- In the event of pronounced dysphagia, it is prudent to administer the anticholinesterase agent parenterally or via a gastric tube, in order to avoid a faux-route [66].
- Start with a low dose, and gradually increase the dose over the day by taking 3 to 6 doses, depending on efficacy, tolerance and duration of action [49] (aiming for the minimum effective dose).
- There is no advantage in combining two cholinesterase inhibitors simultaneously [29].
-Nicotinic and muscarinic side effects should be known to the patient, and are generally less pronounced if taken with a meal, and are dose-dependent, reversible on discontinuation or dosage reduction, or by atropine injection [38].

V.3.1.3 Cholinergic crisis :

-Anticholinesterase agents can occupy the same receptors as acetylcholine, and their excess can depress neuromuscular transmission. The curarizing effect of anticholinesterase agents is a serious therapeutic risk[20].
-The cholinergic crisis shares with the myasthenic crisis a rapid motor and respiratory deterioration. It is characterized by Signs of cholinergic overdose:

- Abundant fasciculations,
- Digestive signs (nausea, vomiting, diarrhea),
- Hyper salivation,
- Bronchial hypersecretion,
- Sweating,
- Watery eyes,
- Pallor,
- Myosis,
- Bradycardia.

It's much rarer than myasthenic crisis, but the two complications can be intertwined.

V.3.2. Background treatment :

V.3.2.1 Long-term immunotherapy :

Immunosuppressive drugs address the cause of the pathology by limiting immune system hyperreactivity [39,63, 51].
Since they are taken on a long-term basis and can have potentially significant side-effects, these drugs are only proposed as second-line treatment when symptoms are not sufficiently or durably improved by anticholinesterase agents, and will need to be closely monitored.
Since immunosuppression is not selective, and the adverse effects can be serious, the benefit-risk balance will enable a choice to be made between the various options currently available.
These treatments are mainly indicated in cases of generalized myasthenia.
The majority of recommendations concerning the prescription of immunosuppressive agents are not based on large-scale, prospective, double-blind, randomized controlled trials. They are based either on randomized controlled trials involving small numbers of patients, or simply on anecdotal evidence [38].
Because they reduce the immune system's defenses, a pre-existing infectious problem (viral or bacterial) must be ruled out before starting them, with particular attention paid to tuberculosis [29].

Side effects common to most immunosuppressants
-Increased risk of infection
-Increased risk of malignant tumors.

Things to remember for the patient:
-Watch out for any fever or signs of infection and seek medical advice.
-Live vaccines are not recommended, or even contraindicated, as there is a risk of generalized vaccine disease.
Regular monitoring of tumor markers and radiological follow-up.
-This is background treatment, so in the event of acute worsening of the pathology, there's no need to increase doses.

-Longer or shorter duration of action (several weeks to several months): do not stop if there is no rapid improvement [68].

V.3.2.1.1 First-line treatment :

It is based on either corticosteroids or Azathioprine (Imurel®), or a combination of the two. Mycophenolatemofetyl (Cellcept®) is an alternative to Azathioprine. The choice of treatment depends on the time to onset of action, contraindications and sometimes the patient's wishes [29].

❖ **Corticosteroid therapy (glucocorticoids):**

Known for their beneficial effects in many other autoimmune diseases, they are the oldest disease-modifying therapy for myasthenia gravis [38,64], used as initial immunotherapy [37] and the most widely used [38,64], although there are very few controlled studies to date in this indication.

➢ **Indication:**

Indicated in generalized myasthenia that responds poorly to symptomatic treatment [37,49] and in the absence of contraindications [49].

To improve muscle strength or in preparation for thymectomy [20]. Rarely in pure ocular myasthenia when diplopia is troublesome [20]. It is beneficial in 75% of cases. Improvement occurs 2 to 4 weeks after the start of treatment [29,49].

There is some evidence to suggest that this therapeutic class may also delay or limit the progression of pure ocular myasthenia to generalized myasthenia [38].

➢ **Administration**

Prednisone (cortancyl°) and prednisolone (solupred°) are the most commonly used corticoids. Treatment modalities vary from author to author. Oral absorption of prednisone is rapid[69].

In generalized myasthenia, the usual initial treatment is 1 mg/kg/day of prednisone or prednisolone (60-100mg per day)[29] .

This dose can lead to an increase in muscle weakness [20], and thus the occurrence of transient worsening of symptoms [29] (in 50% of cases [49]) during the first 15 days on corticosteroids is frequent and worrying, especially when the myasthenia is already severe (risk of myasthenic crisis) [29]. This justifies initial hospitalization to initiate treatment [29,49], at best close to an intensive care unit. To avoid this initial aggravation, it has been suggested that treatment should be started at lower doses [29,70], of the order of 15 to 25 mg, and increased in stages.

This gradual increase has the disadvantage of delaying the effect of treatment [70] (a low dose leads to improvement only after 2 months [20]).

To avoid this aggravation while maintaining a short onset of action, patients with swallowing or respiratory disorders may be given a combination of EP or IV IG during the first week of corticosteroid therapy.

The dosage of 1mg/kg/d is usually continued for 1 month or until improvement is achieved.

The dosage is then reduced by 10 mg/month to 0.5mg/kg/d, then by 5 mg/month to reach a plateau of around 10 mg/d [71]. Maintenance doses are then continued [20].

In principle, corticosteroids should only be reduced once significant improvement has been achieved (MGFA class II minimal manifestations).
Dosage reduction should always be gradual, and complete cessation should never take place before one year's treatment.
At the slightest sign of recurrence, the dosage reduction should be continued and, if necessary, the dosage increased again [29].
In some patients, maintenance treatment can be discontinued without the clinical symptoms reappearing [20].
With the aim of reducing the side effects of corticosteroid therapy, many authors, particularly in the USA, prescribe higher doses, but alternating every other day [20,70].
According to the majority of authors, the results of corticosteroid therapy are good or very good. The percentage of remission and significant improvement in four series, each involving more than 60 patients, ranges from 72% to 92% [72,73,74,75].
Improvement is rapid, appearing between 1 and 21 days in over 85% of patients [73,74]. Maximum results are achieved within 6 [101,102,103] or 12 months [75].
In most cases, treatment has to be continued at a reduced but variable dosage for several years to maintain improvement; only 5 to 14% of patients in the four series were able to be totally free of corticosteroids.
Arsura[120] proposed very high-dose corticosteroids for the treatment of myasthenic crises.
The side effects of long-term corticosteroid therapy are significant in all series, affecting 38% to 67% of patients [66].
Long-term maintenance of low-dose corticosteroids is often necessary to avoid symptom relapse, which implies a significantly increased risk of adverse effects [37,38].
As these undesirable effects can become limiting for a significant number of patients, this has necessitated the introduction of other immunosuppressive agents in myasthenia gravis: "cortisone-sparing immunosuppressive agents", which can either replace corticosteroid therapy, or be combined with it to reduce the dose of prednisone/prednisolone as much as possible [76].

❖ **Cytotoxic immunosuppressants :**

Treatment with cytotoxic immunosuppressants (IS) was proposed as early as 1967 [71]. Azathioprine is the most widely used drug, and is indicated when the disease is resistant to corticosteroids alone, or when corticosteroids are contraindicated.

o **Azathioprine (Imurel°)**

➢ **Indication**

Initially indicated mainly for the prevention of transplant rejection, it is the main non-steroidal immunosuppressive agent prescribed for autoimmune myasthenia gravis. It is a cytotoxic agent [77].

➢ **Administration**

The initial dose is 2 to 3 mg/kg/day. The onset of action averages 3 to 6 months [38,49, 64].
According to retrospective studies in myasthenia, its efficacy is similar to that of corticosteroids (over 70% clinical improvement), but its onset of action is much longer.

It takes 2 to 10 months to see an improvement in muscle strength, and the maximum benefit is therefore delayed compared with corticosteroids [38,64].
However, its safety profile is more favorable.
Discontinuation should be considered over the long term (minimum 5 years) to limit the risk of relapse, and after at least 12 to 18 months at the maximum dose.
This drug was the first to prove its cortisone-sparing effect, and it was also shown that patients had longer remissions, fewer relapses and fewer adverse drug reactions than with corticosteroid therapy alone [64].
Imurel® is indicated as a long-term immunosuppressant in myasthenia gravis, either as a cortisone-sparing agent (to reduce the dosage of glucocorticoids) or as first-line immunotherapy if time to onset is not a limiting factor [37].
It significantly reduces the dose of corticosteroids and is therefore often used in combination with them.
The occurrence within the first few days of a febrile syndrome with asthenia, digestive disorders or skin rash, indicating an allergic reaction, requires definitive discontinuation of treatment.
More frequently, chronic cases of leukopenia, thrombocythemia and impaired liver function occur; azathioprine must be reduced or sometimes discontinued, and then gradually reintroduced if biological parameters return to normal.
Exceptional cases of pancreatitis have also been described.
It is recommended that Azathioprine treatment be discontinued only after several years of satisfactory control, to limit the risk of relapse [29].
In cases of resistance to Imurel® or corticosteroids alone, their combination is often effective [49]. Imurel® is taken in 1 to 3 doses during the day, at mealtimes [68].

- **Mycophenolatemofetil (Cellcept°)**

Another anti-metabolite cytotoxic agent, this relatively recent immunosuppressive agent selectively inhibits purine synthesis in B and T lymphocytes, thus blocking their proliferation in a manner quite similar to azathioprine [37,38].

➢ **Indication**

Initially used to prevent transplant rejection, like azathioprine, this molecule has shown minimal toxicity, making it suitable for long-term use in myasthenia gravis, as a cortisone-sparing agent or as immunotherapy alone in cases of contraindication or significant iatrogenicity with subcorticoids.
As with azathioprine, improvement in muscle strength appears to be delayed by at least two months compared with treatment initiation.
This drug is still recommended as a second-line immunosuppressive therapy in cases of myasthenia refractory to previous treatments, or in cases of contraindications to these drugs [78].

➢ **Administration**

The recommended dosage is 2 g/day in two doses. Tolerance is generally good (fewer side effects than azathioprine), but the gain in efficacy over azathioprine is often disappointing.
As with azathioprine, treatment should be discontinued only after several years of stabilization [36].

V.3.2.1.2 Second-line treatments

These are used when previous treatments have failed to control myasthenia or have been poorly tolerated.
The choice of treatment depends on the severity of the clinical picture, the terrain, the time it takes for the various treatments to take effect and their side effects, all of which need to be taken into consideration. Advice from a reference center is essential.
None of the second-line treatments has demonstrated superiority, and in all cases their efficacy needs to be assessed over 9 to 12 months [29].

- **Rituximab (Mabthéra ®)**

This is a genetically-modified chimeric mouse/human monoclonal antibody representing a glycosylated immunoglobulin with human IgG1 constant regions and variable light and heavy chainmurine region sequences.
The antibody is produced by a suspension culture of mammalian cells (Chinese hamster). It is approved for the treatment of certain types of lymphoma and severe active rheumatoid arthritis in adults who have had an inadequate or intolerant response to other disease-modifying anti-rheumatic drugs.
Rituximab binds specifically to the transmembrane antigen CD20, a nonglycosylated phosphoprotein localized on pre-B and mature B lymphocytes.
CD20 is found on normal and malignant B cells, but not on hematopoietic stem cells, pro-B cells, normal plasma cells or other normal tissues.
Toxicity studies have shown no effects other than the expected pharmacological depletion of B cells in peripheral blood and lymphoid tissue. Peripheral B-cell counts are below normal after the first dose of rituximab. Reappearance of B lymphocytes begins within 6 months of the return to normal levels between 9 and 12 months after the end of treatment.
Rituximab offers promising prospects for the treatment of MG, although no randomized controlled trials have been conducted to date.
Case reports, retrospective small series and uncontrolled studies describe a pronounced and prolonged clinical benefit from rituximab, even in patients with severe MG.
More interestingly, it may give better clinical benefit and last longer in anti-MuSK patients than inanti-AChR MG [113].case observation studies have reported its efficacy in refractory generalized myasthenia gravis, as well as a good tolerability profile [65].it is currently proposed in forms resistant to corticosteroids and azathioprine.
Its cost is high, but results are good in some patients, both in classic seropositive forms and in those with anti-MuSK antibodies.
The proposed dose is 375 mg/m2 per week by intravenous infusion, four weeks in succession, or 1 g twice (15 days apart). The prevention of severe allergic reactions requires a preventive protocol of solumedrol and antihistamines prior to Rituximab injection. Repeat courses of Rituximab should be discussed in the light of progress.
Complications are rare, but prior or concomitant immunosuppressive therapy increases the risk of opportunistic infection[29].

- **Etanercept (Enbrel®)**

FC recombinant soluble TNF-alpha receptor has sometimes been used in this autoimmune disease.
A few studies seem to show efficacy on myasthenic symptoms, but their number and quality are insufficient [78].

❖ **Ciclosporin (Neoral ®), and Tacrolimus (Prograf®, Advagraf LP®)**
These molecules have improved myasthenia refractory to other treatments, but they require close monitoring and adaptation of therapy due to their serious side effects [29].

V.3.3. Management of myasthenic attacks Short-term immunotherapy :

It is based on two different therapeutic strategies: plasmapheresis (or plasma exchange) and intravenous human immunoglobulin (Tegelins®).
However, they share the same indications, namely the acute management of exacerbations or myasthenic crises. Both techniques can also be used to prepare myasthenic patients for thymectomy or other surgical procedures [29,49, 64].
Similarly, their use at the start of treatment with corticosteroids to prevent or limit cortico-induced exacerbations [37,49,113], as well as their prescription as monotherapy for rare patients refractory to all other forms of treatment, are among the possible indications for these short-term immunosuppressive treatments, indications supported by an official NIH (National Institute of Health) consensus dating from 1986 [37,113].
They can improve muscle strength, but only temporarily, over a period of a few weeks: they therefore require the administration of long-acting immunomodulatory agents to manage the underlying pathological phenomenon [49,51].
As these treatments are prescribed and used almost exclusively in the hospital setting, they will not be developed further here [66]. PE and IVIg have similar efficacy, but some patients respond preferentially to one or the other therapy.

The choice between IVIg and PE depends on their respective contraindications and what the hospital can offer, especially for PE.

Headache is not uncommon with IVIG, lasting from a few hours to a few days, and improving with analgesics and rest. Rare observations of aseptic meningitis have been reported. [29]

V.3.3.1 Plasma exchange (PE)

Plasma exchanges will allow transient elimination of circulating antibodies, including anti-RACh [64].
Improvement occurs within a few days in most patients, usually after the second or third exchange session [37,38].
Antibody levels generally fall by 75% after treatment, but will rise again fairly rapidly, as early as two weeks after the end of treatment [67]. The number of exchanges and the time between exchanges will depend on severity and response: from 2 to 4, on average over one to 3 weeks [29].
Clinical benefit never lasts more than 4 to 10 weeks [76].

V.3.3.2 Intravenous immunoglobulins :

Initially used in many autoimmune diseases, IV immunoglobulins have a much more complex mechanism [38].
Their efficacy in improving the symptoms of myasthenia has been demonstrated in a placebo-controlled study [119]. The time to clinical improvement is quite variable (one to two weeks) and can take up to 19 days [37].
The use of IVIg was proposed as early as 1984 [79].
Since then, several open studies have reported favorable results using infusions of 0.4 g/kg/d of IgG for 5 days [80] (2g/Kg), but the number of infusions can be reduced to2(1g/Kg per infusion).

Improvement is maximal between the 15th and 25th day after the start of treatment. Side effects of IGIV, of the order of 5%, are generally minor, but anaphylactic shock, aseptic meningitis and acute renal failure have been reported, and the risk of transmission of infectious agents must be borne in mind.IGIVs are contraindicated in cases of severe renal impairment, high and uncontrolled thromboembolic risk, and IgA deficiency.

The immunomodulatory effects of polyvalent IVIg depend on several mechanisms of action, which differ according to the autoimmune pathology involved. Neutralization of circulating pathogenic autoantibodies by autoantibody-idiotype interaction is responsible for a rapid decrease in autoantibody titer.
IVIg also contains antibody specificities directed against numerous lymphocyte surface molecules involved in the regulation of immune responses, which account for the long-term effects of IVIg administration [66].
This surgical procedure is part of the standard therapeutic arsenal for the autoimmune pathology we are studying, but its effect is not immediate, and clinical benefit may not be observed until several months or even years later [37, 40, 49].
In 15% of cases, myasthenia gravis is associated with a tumour of the thymus; this is the formal indication for thymectomy; it is generally a case of severe, late-onset myasthenia gravis, with no gender predominance. Removal may be supplemented by radiotherapy or even chemotherapy, depending on the histological findings [64].

V.3.4 Other treatments

-The value of psychological treatment must be assessed according to the patient's needs. patients and during their evolution.
First-line analgesics (paracetamol) and massage are useful in cases of pain secondary to spinal muscle weakness, particularly neck pain caused by weak neck extensors.
- Physiotherapy involving retraining and strength training is contraindicated in myasthenic patients.
- On the other hand, the gradual resumption of physical activity (walking, cycling) is a good idea.
desirable to combat the de-training effect of illness [20].

VI. Practical initiation of treatment :

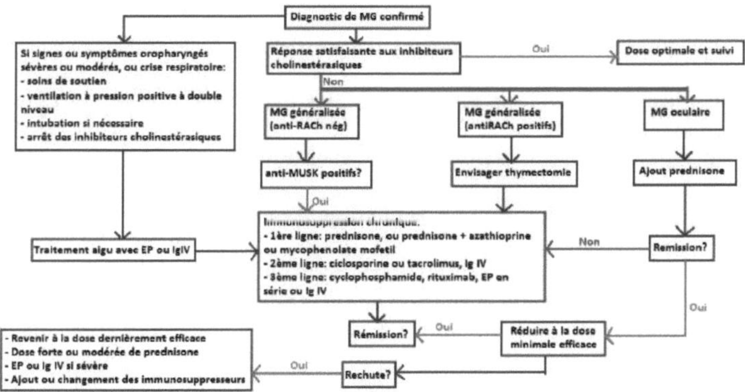

VI.1 Adjusting treatments to disease progression :

The need for anticholinesterase treatment may vary from one period to the next.
the other. Dosage may be reduced spontaneously or after initiation of immunomodulatory therapy, or increased in the event of a demyasthenic flare-up.
Dosages must be adapted to prevent under- and overdosing, which can sometimes lead to motor failure.
In principle, corticosteroid therapy should only be reduced once significant improvement has been achieved (minimal MGFA class II manifestations), and azathioprine or mycophenolatemofetyl should only be discontinued after several years of satisfactory control to limit the risk of relapse.
In fact, many patients require prolonged treatment with corticosteroids and/or immunosuppressants (for 5 to 10 years, and in some cases permanently).
Myasthenia refractory to first-line immunomodulatory treatments should be referred to a Reference Center.
It is important to check that the patient is suffering from myasthenia gravis, that the severity of the disease has been confirmed, and that the patient's previous treatment regimen was correct in terms of the molecules used, the duration and timing of administration, and the patient's discipline/compliance with treatment.
An aggravating factor must be sought: contraindicated medication, associated autoimmune disease.
In some patients, regular (monthly) PE or IVIg may be necessary as background therapy (in case of intolerance or ineffectiveness of other treatments) [29].

VI.2Acute flare-up of myasthenia :

This is a life-saving emergency. The patient's respiratory function must be preserved.

Thrust management proceeds as follows:
-stop all food intake, even liquids by mouth, because of the danger of a false stomach.
-intravenous infusion.
-intramuscular or intravenous injection of 1 mg neostigmine, to be repeated as required a few minutes later.
-intramuscular injection of 0.25 mg atropine to limit hypersecretion in the mouth and bronchi favored by prostigmine.
-oxygen therapy via nasal tube, mask or manual respirator.
-Aspiration of nasopharyngeal secretions.
-medical transport of the patient, as soon as possible, to a medical service resuscitation.
-continuation of anticholinesterase treatment with crushed tablets to be administered by stomach tube, in divided doses and with a moderate dosage.

If there is any doubt as to the nature of the myasthenic or cholinergic crisis, it is best to discontinue the anticholinesterase agents, as the patient is safe from the moment he is intubated and ventilated. If the myasthenic crisis persists, recourse may be had to :
-IV infusion of gamma globulin at a dose of 0.4 g/Kg/24h for 5 hours.
days: this therapy has the advantage of simplicity, and is an alternative to to plasma exchange. Favourable results are observed in around 50% of cases.
-Plasma exchange (plasmapheresis): lowers acetylcholine receptor antibody levels, with no formal clinical correlation.
They are mainly used in severe forms, preoperatively, before lathymectomy [20]; each series comprises 3 to 5 sessions.

Because of the temporary action of plasma exchanges, it is necessary to combine them with a unosuppressive treatment: prednisone (1 mg/Kg/24h) alone or combined with azathioprine (2mg/Kg/24h).

PRACTICAL INFORMATION

I. Introduction - Issues :

Myasthenia gravis (MG) is an autoimmune disease of the neuromuscular junction, preferentially affecting young women and the elderly, with an increasing incidence. Remissions and exacerbations are typical. The disease is caused by autoantibodies directed against acetylcholine receptors or, more rarely, against a muscle-specific kinase. The main therapeutic objective is remission, which is achieved through ongoing collaboration between the treating physician and the patient, and the combination of symptomatic drugs (anticholinesterase agents) and immunomodulators/suppressants (prednisone and azathioprine), or even other alternative treatments.

The diagnosis of myasthenia gravis is often not easy to make, given the clinical polymorphism that it can take on. It is evoked after a careful clinical examination, confirmed by a series of complementary examinations, an anti-acetyl choline receptor antibody assay, an ENMG that highlights a decrement, a thoracic CT scan in search of a thymoma.

A therapeutic test with anti-esterase choline confirms the diagnosis after rapid improvement of clinical signs.

II. Clinical cases

We report the case of patient F.F, aged 37, from and living inMostaganem, admitted on 13/12/2022 to the medical resuscitation department of CHU Mostaganem for management of acute respiratory distress.

The patient is married, mother of 3 G3P3 children, including 2 caesarean sections; her children are alive and well. She has been asthmatic since 2002, unbalanced with 2 hospitalizations in the pneumology department, the first in 2006 for severe acute asthma and the second in 2017 for pneumonia.psoriasisconcomitant with asthmatic disease in 2002. In 2016, on the occasion of a systematic check-up, the diagnosis of right thyroid micronodules was made, with a thyroid work-up disturbed on several occasions. Active temporal epilepsy with left meso-limbic sclerosis diagnosed in April 2021 treated with

Lamotrigine 50mg, 1 cp in the morning and gardenal 100 mg (1 cp and ¼) in the evening. She presented with Algie vasculaire de la face in 2021 treated with 02 sessions.Lastly in October 2022 myasthenia was diagnosed.

Discovery and evolution of the patient's chronic diseases:

We'll start with the discovery of asthma, which began in August 2002. The patient presented with attacks of asthma and a dry cough for over 1 month, with the onset of pulmonary sibilants, respiratory discomfort and orthopnea, bronchial asthma was diagnosed, and treatment with inhaled corticosteroids, short-acting bronchodilators, long-acting bronchodilators, antibiotics and oral corticosteroids was prescribed. Allergological tests were carried out, with strongly positive results for dust and house dust mites.

From 2002 to 2017, the respiratory symptomatology was marked by two hospitalizations in the pneumology department of CHU Oran. The first was in 2006 for 5 days for severe acute asthma, treated with Celestenecompressed oral corticosteroids for 1 month, with side effects such as facial acne and weight gain of 20 kg, which prompted the patient to discontinue treatment abruptly. The second in 2017 for 15 days for community-acquired pneumonia treated with antibiotics and corticosteroids.

In 2013, her first pregnancy was a difficult twin with EUS of one of the two fetuses, and survival of the second with a dystocic delivery requiring the use of forceps. Postpartum, the patient presented with significant asthenia and a worsening of her asthmatic pathology.

In 2016, she gave birth to her second child after a difficult pregnancy. She underwent caesarean section under general anaesthesia. Our patient gave birth to a newborn with a cleft lip. Postoperatively, she experienced drowsiness for 48 hours, followed by dizziness, muscle fatigue and an inability to stand for 1 week. Subsequently, our patient began to develop daytime absences with amnesia, muscular fatigue on exertion and unilateral ptosis at first, then bilateral.

Given this symptomatology, the diagnosis of post-partum depression was made, and the patient was treated with an antidepressant such as Depretine 20 mg daily and a benzodiazepine such as Kietyl. This treatment was maintained for 1 year, despite worsening neurological signs (muscle fatigue and ptosis). The decrease in visual acuity at the end of the day prompted the doctors to refer the patient to an ophthalmologist, who prescribed vision correction.

The improvement of respiratory and neurological signs by the corticosteroid therapy prescribed for the management of her asthma led the patient to self-medicate with this molecule.

In 2019, the 3rd pregnancy was more difficult than the previous ones, requiring 9 months off work. Our patient benefited from a caesarean section performed under spinal anaesthesia. In the immediate post-partum period, she presented with generalized tonic-clonic seizures treated with benzodiazepine, with intense muscle fatigue and an inability to stand.

During the same year, neurological symptoms progressed steadily, with muscular fatigue on exertion and limitation of daily activities, difficulty of speech, nasal voice, ptosis and visual disturbances with periods of remission.

In April 2021, the patient presented with a generalized tonic-clonic seizure, treated urgently with valium enIV, prompting an EEGobjective of active temporal epilepsy and a brain MRI showing hypocampal-right sclerosis.

The patient was started on tegretol 400mg, replaced by Keppra 500mg and then 750mg, due to an allergic reaction and the development of inverted psoriasis following this treatment.

The epileptic disease worsening more and more with increased frequency of absences, appearance of myoclonus of the upper and lower limbs with palpebral automatisms (blinking) at a frequency of 8 seizures per day this symptomatology was stabilized in April 2022 under lamotrigine 50 mg and gardenal 100 mg.

In May 2022, a diagnosis of facial vascular pain was made, treated by 15-minute oxygen therapy sessions.

At the end of August 2022, the patient presented with an influenza-like illness, with worsening neurological signs, an increase in the duration of absences to over an hour, worsening muscle fatigue, nasal voice, ptosis, diplopia and the appearance of false routes, prompting her GP to refer her to the neurology department of the CHUOran. In view of this picture, the diagnosis of myasthenia was suspected, justifying the neostigmine test, which came back positive with a spectacular improvement in symptomatology.

An ENMG was ordered, showing a post-synaptic block in favor of a myasthenic syndrome with myogenic involvement. In the light of these clinical and paraclinical arguments, the diagnosis of myasthenia was made as Osserman stage IIa, and treatment with mestinon 60 mg cp every 8 h was administered, with a gradual increase in dose up to the maximum dosage: 1cp/ 4 h in November 2022.

Response to treatment was inadequate. Investigations were completed by a thoracic CT scan for thymoma, which returned unremarkable, and an anti-RAC antibody assay, which returned negative.

Hospitalization in the intensive care unit

On 12/13/2022, the patient was referred to the intensive care unit of Mostaganem University Hospital via the neurology department for management of a myasthenic crisis with acute respiratory distress and swallowing disorder.

On admission, the patient was conscious and uncooperative, scored 14/15 GS, with slurred speech, a blocked voice and bilateral ptosis. Hemodynamic and respiratory status: BP 125/65, tachycardia at 112 beats per minute, polypnea at 23 cycles per minute, SpO2 91%, apyretic at 37.1°C, pulmonary auscultation revealed diffuse bilateral sibilant rales, with inverted psoriasis (inguinal folds) on skin examination.

The patient was hospitalized, with monitoring of : BP ECG FC FR SpO2, oxygen therapy 6 liters, antibiotic therapy based on Augmentin3g/d, solumedrol 40 mg IV, nebulization with salbutamol, rehydration regimen, lovenox 0.4 /24 h with maintenance of her per os trainement: Mestinon 60 mg / 4h with Gardenal and lamotrigine.

Decompensation of myasthenia was suspected, and IV immunoglobulins were indicated. The patient did not receive them because they were not available.

Developments during hospitalization are detailed in the following paragraphs.

- **The week from December 13, 2022 to December 18, 2022:**

During this week, we witnessed several convulsive seizures (more than 10 seizures / 24 h) of the complex partial epilepsy type (absence + myocolonies of the left upper and lower limbs and blink-type palpebral automatisms) lasting less than 2 min. The patient is still myasthenic, with inability to hold her head alone and slowness of speech. The patient benefited from a modification of the anti-acetyl-cholinesterase regimen "mestinon 60mg at 7 a.m./11 a.m./3 p.m./9 p.m./00 p.m." with administration of mestinon LP 180mg at 5 p.m. Antibiotic and corticosteroid therapy were maintained. Biological work-up was normal

Respiratory symptoms improved, with disappearance of pulmonary sibilants and saturation at 95% on room air.

- **The week from December 19, 2022 to December 25, 2022:**

Given the high frequency of convulsive seizures, the patient was transported by the Mostaganem SAMU team to the Mostaganem CHU psychiatry department for an inter-critical EEG, which came back without any particularities.

On December 20, 2022, the patient's condition improved, with the ability to hold her head on her own, good muscle tone, mobilization of the upper limbs with heaviness of the lower limbs. This symptomatology was replaced by ptosis and muscle fatigue at the end of the day. A second test for antibody anti RAC and antiMusket was negative (< 0.1, and < 0.18), Cortisolaemia at 8 a.m. was normal, electrolytes (Ca^+, Na^+, K^+) were normal and thyroid function tests were unremarkable.

Internal medicine was consulted, and an autoimmune polyendocrinopathy was suspected. The following workup was requested: CBC, specific IgE assay, serum protein immunoelectrophoresis, TSH, anti-TPO, anti-thyroglubulin, ANCA, cortisolemia, synacthen test, and a centrifugation sample.

On December 22, 2022, immunoglobulins were finally available and treatment was started at a dose of 0.4g/kg/day, i.e. a total of 30 g per day, 3 vials of 10 mg each lasting 2 hours. 3 days after the start of treatment, the patient experienced adverse effects such as headache, fever peaks, nausea, vomiting, angina pain, metallic taste in the mouth, dyspnoea with chest pain, justifying a reduction in dose to 20g / day, allowing better tolerance of the treatment.

- **The week from December 26, 2022 to December 30, 2022** :

After a 06-day course of immunoglobulin, there was a marked improvement in her neurological condition. The patient was conscious and cooperative, with fluent speech, no ptosis and a reduction in the intensity of muscular fatigue.

She was discharged on 05-01-2023, with discharge treatment: Mestinon 60 mg 7h 11 h 15 h 21 h 00 h MestionLp 180 mg Lamotrigine 50 mg 1 cp in the morning Gardenal 100 mg 1cp and ¼

2 weeks after discharge, the patient presented with abdominal bloating, profuse diarrhea, hyper salivation and sweating. The diagnosis of a cholinergic syndrome was made, treated with atropine , and a therapeutic readjustment was made, Mestinon LP in the morning at 7 a.m. , Mestinon 60 mg at 3 p.m. and at 8 p.m. . This readjustment allowed signs to regress.

III. Discussion:

This case is very interesting, and has enabled us to develop several chapters relating to this pathology.

In summary, we report the case of a 37-year-old woman who began presenting with signs of myasthenia since 2016 and was not diagnosed until late 2022, a total of 07 years after the onset of symptomatology.This case is indicative of the difficulties encountered in making the diagnosis of myasthenia.

In fact, it is a potentially serious chronic neuromuscular disease of autoimmune origin, which can be life-threatening in advanced forms with respiratory involvement. At the beginning, it often manifests itself as fluctuating and reversible ophthalmic signs, such as ptosis, diplopia and visual blur, especially at the end of the day or during exertion, which are consistent with our patient's signs.

The diagnosis was made 7 years after the onset of signs at the stage of generalized muscle fatigue with bulbar and respiratory signs, corresponding to stage IIa in Osserman's classification.

1. Diagnosis of myasthenia :

The positive diagnosis was made in 2022 on the basis of a number of clinical and para-clinical arguments:

- The presence of suggestive signs and symptoms since 2016: diplopia, visual blur, ptosis, without pupillary anomaly, bulbar disorders (nasal voice, false routes, chewing and/or lingual motor disorders), weakness and fatigue of the limbs and cervical muscles (inability to hold the head alone); the exclusively muscular nature (no sensory disorders, no central or peripheral neurological impairment, no signs of dysautonomia).

-Aggravation by effort (e.g. nasation after a long discussion). Other aggravating factors in this case were: antidepressant, antiepileptic treatment, pregnancy and post-partum, infectious episodes.

- A specific chronology with symptom variability: fluctuating during the day (increased in the evening or when exerting oneself), or part of an unexpected flare-up, corresponding to a worsening of the disease over a period of several weeks to several months.
- Further investigations: ENMG in October 2022: showed decrement and post-synaptic block in favour of a myasthenic syndrome with myogenic involvement. Cervical CT scan showed no thymoma.
- Response was favorable to anti-cholinesterase agents
- Antibody ani ACH negative anti Musk negative concluded seronegative myasthenia.

2. Seronegative myasthenia :

Anti-acetyl choline antibodies are positive in 85% of patients with generalized myasthenia**[11]**.

However, in our case, the myasthenia is seronegative, as shown by the antibody assays (anti Rach/ antiMusk repeated 2 times with a 4-month interval).we speak of seronegative myasthenia if the anti-acetyl choline receptor antibodies are negative, involving other antibodies, i.e. myasthenias associated with anti-MuSK, low-affinity antiRACh and anti-LRP4 antibodies.

Anti-MuSK seronegative myasthenias are characterized by a high preponderance of females of all ages, generalized myasthenia gravis, marked severity with significant bulbar and respiratory involvement, requiring immunosuppressive treatment, associated with thymic involution, or absence of thymoma. The disappointing response to anticholinesterase drugs and the frequent negativity of electroneuromyographic exploration (absence of decrement) complicate the diagnosis[**10**].

Myasthenias associated with low-affinity anti-RACh and anti-LRP4 antibodies are similar to those of classical myasthenia with anti-RACh antibodies: preponderance of females, usually involved in generalized forms[**10**].

In 40% of generalized myasthenias without anti-RACh, antibodies directed against another post-synaptic anti-MuSK molecule are detected. For generalized myasthenia without anti-RACh or anti-MuSK antibodies, known as seronegative myasthenia, two categories of antibodies have recently been described using immunostaining techniques on HEK (Human Embryonic Kidney) cells: low-affinity anti-RACh antibodies and anti-LRP4 antibodies (LRP4 is the receptor for agrin, which activates MuSK). The assay of these antibodies is not yet routinely available[**10**].

3. Myasthenic crisis:

The evolution of myasthenia gravis is marked in most cases by episodes of worsening of the deficit signs, especially during the first years of the disease's evolution , when episodes of exacerbation are common, and can be severe, requiring resuscitation.

The Myasthenia Gravis Foundation of America (MGFA) clinical classification is intended to identify MG subgroups with different clinical signs or severity: [11]

- Class I: eye muscle deficit. May have weakness of eye occlusion. The strength of all other muscles is normal;
- Class II: Discrete deficit of muscles other than the ocular muscles. May have ocular muscle deficits of any severity:
    - IIa: predominantly affecting limb or axial muscles;
    - IIb: predominantly affecting oropharyngeal or respiratory muscles;

- Class III: moderate deficit of muscles other than ocular muscles. May have ocular muscle deficits of any severity:
  - IIIa: predominantly affecting limb or axial muscles;
  - IIIb: predominantly affecting oropharyngeal or respiratory muscles;
- Class IV: severe deficit of muscles other than ocular muscles. May have ocular muscle deficit of any severity:
- IVa: predominantly affecting limb or axial muscles;
- IVb: predominantly affecting oropharyngeal or respiratory muscles
- Class V: need for intubation.

Certain events likely to have favoured the onset of myasthenic decompensation are worth mentioning:**[12]**

- Surgery, particularly if curares have been used. Myasthenic crises have been observed after removal of a thymoma that appeared isolated preoperatively (15-20% of myasthenias are accompanied by a thymic tumor);
- Infections such as pneumonia, frequently the cause of myasthenic decompensation, can also be a consequence of inhalation;
- Treatment likely to alter neuromuscular transmission. Numerous drugs have been incriminated, with varying degrees of imputability: cardiotropics (beta-blockers, calcium channel blockers, class 1 antiarrhythmics), antibiotics (aminoglycosides, polymyxins, injectable cyclins, telithromycin, fluoroquinolones), antimalarials (quinine and related compounds), antiepileptics (phenytoin, carbamazepine), neuroleptics, botulinum toxin, iodinated contrast media, etc.
- During pregnancy, the most critical periods are the first trimester and especially the post-partum period.

The patient presented signs of a severe myasthenic crisis with acute respiratory distress, swallowing disorders and a generalized motor deficit classified III b in MGFA, requiring resuscitation.

4. Myasthenia gravis and pregnancy:

Pregnancy was always a revealing and aggravating factor in the disease, and several studies were carried out on the evolution of myasthenia during pregnancy, childbirth and the post-partum period.

The evolution of myasthenia is variable and unpredictable during pregnancy, was the conclusion of a study published by (CAMBRIDGE UNIVERSITY PRESS ON BEHALF OF THE CANADIAN JOURNAL OF NEUROLOGICAL SCIENCES), which was carried out on 20 myasthenic women, with a total of 28 pregnancies during the period from 2001 to 2019 . The worsening of the women's state of health was observed in 50% of cases , 18% during pregnancy ,25% after childbirth, and 7% from the two previous periods . **[2]**

Table 1: Demographic data on patients with MG and pregnancy

Twenty-eight pregnancies in 20 women	2001–2019
Generalized MG	20 (100)
AChRAb	13 (77)
MuSK	1 (8)
Mean age at the first pregnancy (Y)	29.7 ± 5.7
Mean duration MG (Y)	5.7 ± 5.9
MG worse	16 (57)
MG worse during pregnancy	7 (25)
MG worsening during pregnancy when duration < 2Y	5 (71)
Odds ratio of getting worse with < 2Y MG duration	3.43:1
MG worse after delivery	9 (32)
MG worse when immunosuppression stopped	3 (100)
Onset MG during pregnancy	1 (5)
Onset MG following delivery	1 (5)

AChRAb = acetylcholine receptor antibody; MuSK = muscle specific kinase antibody, Y = years.
Data are given as *n* (%) or as means ± standard deviation.

Another study published in March 2018, carried out on a group of 09 myasthenic women between the ages of 24-35, entitled Myasthenia and pregnancy, whose results were in favor of 56% of women worsening during pregnancy while 44% remained stable, with no improvement observed . On postpartum, 22% worsened, 78% remained stable, with no improvement noted. **[3]**

A third study, based on a retrospective analysis of the files of 100 patients treated for autoimmune myasthenia between 1994 and 2003 in the neurology departments of the Lille CHRU, concluded that 26% of patients had worsened, i.e. 71.4% during the 1st trimester, 59.2% were stable and 4.8% had improved. **[4]**

Tableau V. – Évolution de la myasthénie auto-immune chez les patientes qui ont mené leur grossesse à terme.
Evolution of myasthenia gravis in patients who completed pregnancy.

Évolution de la MAI (n = 27)	Nombre	Pourcentage
Durant la grossesse :		
– amélioration	4	14,8
– stabilisation	16	59,2
– aggravation	7	26
Durant le post-partum :		
– amélioration	2	7,4
– stabilisation	21	77,8
– aggravation	4	14,8

n : nombre de grossesses menées à terme.

Tableau VI. – Modalités des accouchements.
Mode of deliveries.

Paramètres	Nombre (n = 27)	Pourcentage
Voies basses sans forceps	14	52
Voies basses avec forceps	6	22
Césarienne	7	26
Péridurale	18	66,7
Induction du travail (ocytociques)*	10	50
Complications	0	0

*n : nombre de grossesses menées à terme ; * : réalisée sur les accouchements par voies basses.*

For delivery modalities, epidural anesthesia was used in 66.7% of patients , 30% required an instrumental forceps maneuver after prolonged labor , and oxytocin injection in 50% of patients , with 26% of cesarean sections indicated on pure obstetric grounds and have no associations with worsening myasthenia .

In the postpartum period, 4 out of 27 patients worsened, with a single death 1 month after delivery due to respiratory decompensation.

The conclusion of all these studies confirms the unpredictable nature of the evolution of myasthenia during pregnancy. [**4**]

5. Myasthenia gravis and epilepsy:

The association of myasthenia and epilepsy is exceptional. The incidence of epilepsy is 5 to 7 times higher in myasthenics than in the general population. Myasthenia is often associated with other conditions, most of which have an immunological origin; but for the association of myasthenia and epilepsy, the hypotheses explaining such an association are still uncertain. [**5**] ,

For Osserman1958, the association is as exceptional as it is fortuitous; for some, there is a relationship between the two, as myasthenia is more common in epileptics than in the general population, according to several studies. Indeed, Hoefer et al. (1958) reported eight cases of such an association out of a total of 180 myasthenics, representing a frequency of 5%[6] . Rodriguez et al (1983) reported 4 patients with associated epilepsy in a series of 149 patients with juvenile myasthenia**[7]**. Badurska et al (1991) found 8 epileptics among 119 myasthenic children, i.e. 7%**[8] .**

The relationship between the two conditions is as yet unknown, but there is a notion of therapeutic interference: the action of antiepileptic drugs on myasthenia is quite obvious, as in the case of diazepines or carbamazepine. An example of this was reported by Peterson in 1966, who treated petit mal with trimetadione developed a myastheniform syndrome with positive anti-nuclear and anti-muscle antibodies[9]. On the other hand, antimyasthenics have little effect on epilepsy, but plasmapheresis, recognized as an effective treatment for myasthenia, significantly reduces phenytoin concentration and can lead to convulsions.

The association of myasthenia and epilepsy is rare, if not exceptional. Epilepsy is more common in myasthenics than in the general population. This means that a choice of treatment must be made to avoid aggravation of either condition. The mechanism is still unclear.

6. Management of myasthenia :

Our patient received symptomatic, crisis and background treatment.

- **Symptomatic treatment:**

Anticholine-esterase drugs form the basis of the disease's symptomatic treatment. Their use in myasthenia was introduced by Mary Walker in 1934, after she observed an analogy between myasthenic symptoms and those of physostigmine-sensitive curare poisoning (Walker, 1934).(13) By reversibly inhibiting the enzymatic hydrolysis of ACh in the synaptic cleft, anticholinesterase agents prolong the action of the neurotransmitter and thus increase the number of its interactions with the remaining RACh. **[14]**

Two oral anticholinesterase agents are available: pyridostigmine bromide (Mestinon1) and ambenonium chloride (Mytelase1). With an onset of action of 30 minutes, duration of effect is around four hours. Peak pyridostigmine plasma concentration is delayed when food is taken at the same time. In practice, anticholinesterase titration is progressive, with single doses taken half an hour before meals and at least four hours apart.

There is no advantage in combining two anticholinesterase agents. Mestinon1 has a more favorable side-effect profile. Muscarinic adverse effects (intestinal colic, diarrhea, bronchial hypersecretion, sweating) can be reduced by concomitant use of an atropine. Dosages higher than 480 mg pyridostigmine per 24 hours or 60 mg ambenonium per 24 hours run the risk of cholinergic overdosage. Patients with waking symptoms may benefit from taking the delayed-release form of Mestinon1 (180 mg) at bedtime. [13]

- **Treatment of the crisis :**

Short-term immunotherapy is based on two therapeutic modalities: plasma exchange (PE) and intravenous immunoglobulin (IVIG). PE and IVIg share the same indication, namely short-term control of severe relapses and attacks.

EP acts by transiently purifying circulating antibodies. Their practical application (frequency and number of sessions, volume exchanged at each session) has not been codified. In practice, three EPs are generally performed over the first few days, after which the attitude is largely guided by clinical response and tolerance.

The mechanism of action of IVIg is more complex and multifactorial. Their mode of administration (total dosage, duration of treatment) varies from center to center, ranging from 2 g/kg administered over five days to 1 g/kg administered over one day. A randomized study showed equivalent efficacy and tolerance for two protocols (1 g/kg over one day or 2 g/kg over two days).

PE and IVIg have comparable efficacy in treating relapses, with a lower rate of adverse effects for IVIg. Their onset of action is also comparable, in the order of a few days. In the study conducted, the percentage of responders to PE or IVIG did not exceed 50-60%. The ineffectiveness of one technique does not prejudge the effect of the other on the same patient. In practice, the choice between these two techniques is essentially guided by the contraindications (notably infectious for PE, renal for IVIG) and the conditions for implementation (venous access, availability, cost). The effect of PE and IGIV lasts only a few weeks, necessitating the simultaneous use of a background treatment.

Long-term IVIg (monthly courses, for example) is sometimes used successfully either as monotherapy in previously thymectomized patients, or as supplementary training in certain severe refractory forms of myasthenia gravis.

Adverse reactions to human normal immunoglobulin include (in decreasing order of frequency):

- Chills, headache, dizziness, fever, vomiting, allergic reactions, nausea, arthralgia, low blood pressure and moderate low back pain.
- Reversible hemolytic reactions; particularly in patients with blood types A, B or AB, and (rarely) hemolytic anemia requiring transfusion.

- Rarely, abrupt fall in blood pressure and, in isolated cases, anaphylactic shock, even if the patient has not had a hypersensitivity reaction on previous administration.
- (Rarely) transient skin reactions (including cutaneous lupus erythematosus - frequency undetermined).
- (very rarely) thromboembolic reactions such as myocardial infarction, stroke, pulmonary embolism, deep vein thrombosis.
- Reversible aseptic meningitis.
- Cases of increased serum creatinine levels and/or acute renal failure.
- Cases of post-transfusion acute respiratory distress syndrome (TRALI) [16].

- **Background treatment :**

Corticosteroid therapy is the oldest and most widely used disease-modifying treatment for myasthenia gravis. Its efficacy is widely recognized, improving in at least 80% of patients. The onset of action is rapid (two to four weeks on average), and maximum benefit is achieved in an average of five to six months. Initiation of corticosteroid therapy carries the risk of an initial transient worsening of the condition, up to and including a myasthenic crisis. In a series of 116 patients treated with prednisone 1 mg/kg/day, transient worsening was observed in 48% of subjects. It appeared on average after 4.2 days of treatment (extremes: 1-17 days), and intubation proved necessary in ten patients (8.6%). To limit this risk, it is recommended that patients with generalized myasthenia gravis undergo gradual inpatient treatment (Seybold and Drachmann, 1974). If the situation so requires, treatment can be started at the maximum initial dose, in combination with EP or IVIG. The usual initial dose is 1 mg/kg per day. A gradual reduction in dose is only envisaged once a clear clinical improvement has been achieved. Complete weaning cannot always be achieved. In the series by Pascuzzi et al (1984), only 14% of patients were able to discontinue corticosteroid therapy. The frequency and importance of side-effects (weight gain, diabetes, hypertension, cataracts, osteoporosis, psychic disorders, etc.) are the main limitation of this treatment. In a series of 100 patients followed between 1985 and 1989, complications of corticosteroid therapy occurred in 65% of cases, and led to discontinuation in 10% (Beekman et al., 1997).

- **Immunosuppressant:**Retrospective studies indicate that azathioprine (AZA) improves 70-90% of myasthenic patients: AZA is the first immunosuppressant with a proven cortisone-sparing effect. Patients receiving AZA had fewer relapses, longer remissions and fewer side effects. Regular monitoring of blood counts and liver enzymes is recommended throughout treatment. AZA is prescribed at an initial dose of 2 to 3 mg/kg per day, maintained for 12 to 18 months. Because of the risk of relapse when treatment is stopped, it should be continued at a decreasing dose for at least five years. It can be reintroduced in the event of relapse. Other immunosuppressive agents with proven efficacy in myasthenia gravis are cyclosporine as monotherapy or in combination with corticosteroids, and cyclophosphamide in combination with corticosteroids. Because of their more severe side effects and the precautions required for their use, these immunosuppressants are reserved for patients who are refractory to or intolerant of conventional therapies (prednisone and/or AZA). Several observational studies have reported the efficacy and good tolerance of Rituximab in refractory generalized myasthenia regardless of status[15].

Therapeutic strategy : Rev Med Suisse 2007 ; [17]

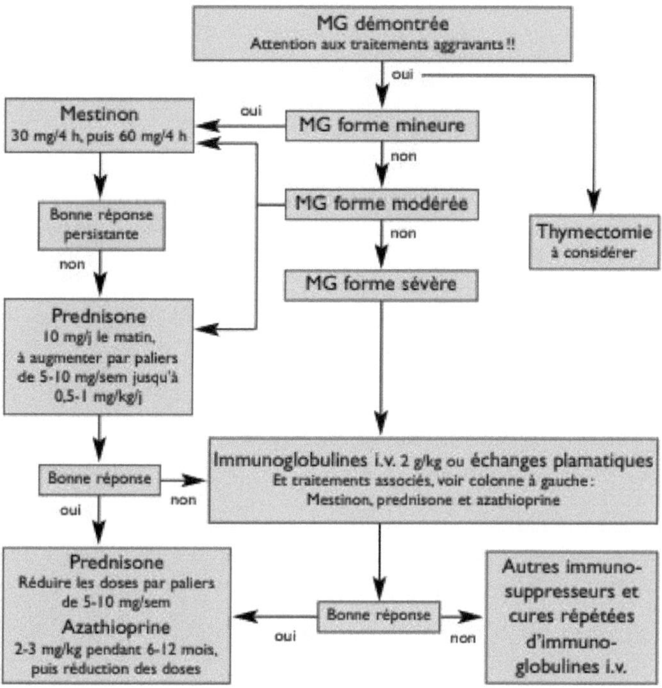

Conclusion:

Autoimmune myasthenia (myasthenia gravis) is a rare disorder of the neuromuscular junction, characterized by muscle weakness in which several muscles are often involved. Occurring at any age, it mainly affects adults under 40, with a female predominance. To date, there is no definitive cure for myasthenia gravis. However, numerous medications are used to reduce symptoms and prevent complications. In most cases, treatment enables sufferers to lead a normal life. Thanks to treatment, mortality has fallen dramatically and has become exceptional in recent years.

Appendices :

Appendix 01: Clinical assessment

1) Motor score (Garches score) maximum 100 points [20].

-Upper limbs extended horizontally in anteposition:

For 150 seconds 15 points.
For 100 seconds 10 points.
For 50 seconds 5 points.

-Lower limbs: patient supine, thighs flexed at 90° to the pelvis, legs at 90° to thighs :

For 75 seconds 15 points.
For 50 seconds 10 points.
For 25 seconds 5 points.

-Head flexion, patient in supine position:

Against resistance 10 points.
Without 5-point resistance.
Impossible 0 points.
-from lying to sitting :

Without the help of but 10 points.
With the help of but 5 points.
Impossible 0 points.

-Extrinsic oculomotricity :

Normal 10 points.
Isolated Ptosis 5 points.
Diplopia 0 points.

-Palpebral occlusion :

Complete 10 points.
Incomplete 5 points.
Tie 0 points.

-mastication :

Normal 10 points.
Decreased 5 points.
Tie 0 points.

-deglutition :

Normal 10 points.

Decreased 5 points.
Tie 0 points.

-phonation :

Normal voice 10 points.
Nasal voice 5 points.
Aphonia 0 points.

2) Daily activity score (over the last 8 days)[29].
An easy-to-use, eight-item questionnaire on activities of daily living has recently been validated:
Elocution: normal 0 / intermittent nasal 1 / permanent 2 / major dysarthria preventing understanding 3

Mastication: normal 0 / fatigue with solid food 1/ fatigue with semiliquid food 2 / nasogastric tube 3

Swallowing: normal 0 / episodic disorders 1 / frequent disorders requiring change of diet 2 / nasogastric tube 3

Respiration: normal 0/exertional dyspnea 1/rest dyspnea 2/ventilation 3

Difficulty brushing or combing teeth: none 0 / effort but without require rest 1 / rest necessary 2 / cannot perform any of these actions 3

Difficulty getting up from a chair: none 0 / sometimes needs help from arms 1 / always needs help from arms 2 / needs assistance 3

Diplopia: none 0 / episodic but not daily 1 / episodic but daily daily 2 / permanent 3

Ptosis: none 0 / episodic but not daily 1 / episodic but daily 2 / permanent 3

Max 24

Appendix 02: Classification of myasthenia gravis severity
A-classification of MGFA [29, 66].
The clinical classification of the Myasthenia Gravis Foundation of America (MGFA) is designed to identify subgroups of MGs with different clinical signs or severity:
- class I: ocular muscle deficit. May have weakness of eye occlusion. The strength of all other muscles is normal;
- class II: discrete deficit of muscles other than the ocular muscles. May have ocular muscle deficits of any severity:
- IIa: predominantly affecting limb or axial muscles;
- IIb: predominantly affecting oropharyngeal or respiratory muscles;
- class III: moderate deficit of muscles other than ocular muscles. May have ocular muscle deficits of any severity:
- IIIa: predominantly affecting limb or axial muscles;
- IIIb: predominantly affecting oropharyngeal or respiratory muscles;

- class IV: severe deficit of muscles other than ocular muscles. May have ocular muscle deficit of any severity:
- IVa: predominantly affecting limb or axial muscles;
- IVb: predominantly affecting oropharyngeal or respiratory muscles;
- class V: need for intubation. The need for a gastric tube alone places the patient in class IV.

B- MGFA post-interventional status [29]
- **Stable complete remission:** no signs or symptoms of myasthenia for at least one year, no treatment
Examination: no weakness, isolated eyelid weakness accepted.
-**Pharmacological remission:** same as 1 except for continued treatment
- **Minimal manifestation: The** patient has no symptoms of limitation.
due to myasthenia, but it has some weaknesses on examination for
some muscles
- **Improved**: A substantial reduction in the symptoms noted before treatment, or a substantial and lasting reduction in the treatment of myasthenia gravis.
- **Unchanged:** No substantial change in clinical manifestations
present prior to treatment or reduction in the treatment of myasthenia gravis
- **Worsening:** Substantial increase in clinical manifestations noted before treatment or increase in myasthenia treatments.
- **Relapse:** The patient has met the criteria for stable complete remission, pharmacological remission or minimal manifestations, but subsequently develops clinical signs beyond those permitted by these criteria.

A- Osserman's classification [20, 42]
This classification, modified by Genkins, has now been abandoned due to its imprecision [51]. Four forms are distinguished:
-Group I: isolated ocular myasthenia gravis [106] (ptosis, diplopia).
-group II A: mild (moderate) generalized myasthenia with ocular and extremity signs, no significant bulbar signs
-group II B: generalized myasthenia of moderate severity, with moderate bulbar and/or oculomotor muscle involvement, variable limb muscle involvement, no seizures.
-group III: fulminant, acute, severe generalized myasthenia gravis, with complications due to severe damage to bulbar and respiratory muscles, necessitating tracheostomy.
Group IV: late-onset generalized myasthenia gravis with bulbar signs and seizures, often the outcome within 2 years of a myasthenia classified in the other groups.

BIBLIOGRAPHIES :

[1] N Satkunam, ZA Siddiqi, D Vethanayagam. Severe asthma associated with myasthenia gravis. Can Respir J 2014;21(1):e1-e3.

[2] Myasthenia Gravis and Pregnancy: Toronto Specialty Center Experience Mohammed Alharbi, Deepak Menon , Carolina Barnett, Hans Katzberg, Mathew Sermer, Vera Bril ABSTRACT

[3] Julien Penvern. Myasthenia and pregnancy: about 9 cases. Sciences du Vivant [q-bio]. 2007. ffhal-01732474

[4] Autoimmune myasthenia gravis and pregnancy: clinical course, delivery and postpartum C. Ramirez1 , J. de Seze1 , O. Delrieu1 , T. Stojkovic1 , S. Delalande1 , F. Fourrier2 , D. Leys1 , L. Defebvre1 , A. Destée1 , P. Vermersch1 1 Clinique Neurologique. 2 Multidisciplinary Intensive Care Unit, Hôpital R. Salengro, CHRU, Lille.

[5]Epilepsy and myasthenia:a case report. M. Grira, S. Benammou, T. Lamouchi, M.S. Harzallah, L. Benslamia, RevNeurol (Paris) 2004; 160: 1, 93-95

[6] Myasthenia Gravis and Epilepsy PAUL F. A. HOEFER, M.D.; HENRY ARANOW Jr, M.D., and LEWIS P. ROWLAND, M.D., New York

[7] RODRIGUEZ M, GOMEZ MR, HOWARD FM JR, TAYLOR WF. (1983). Myasthenia gravis in children: long-term follow-up. Ann Neurol, 13: 504-510.

[8] BADURSKA B, RYNIEWICZ B, KOWALSKI J. (1991). Epileptic seizures in children with myasthenia gravis. Neurol Neurochir Pol, 25: 326-31.

[9] PETERSON H. (1966). Association of trimethadione therapy and myasthenia gravis. N Engl J Med, 274: 566-567

[10] Protocole National de Diagnostic et de Soins (PNDS) Autoimmune myasthenia Text of the PNDS Centre de références de pathologie neuromusculaire Paris Est July 2015

[11] Vincent A, Palace J, Hilton-Jones D. Myasthenia gravis. Lancet 2001;357:2122-8.

[12] How to recognize and treat severe inaugural myasthenic exacerbation? B. Clair Service de réanimation médicale, Hôpital Raymond-Poincaré, 104, boulevard Raymond-Poincaré, 92380 Garches, France

[13] Traitement de la myasthe'nie auto-immune Treatment of autoimmunemyasthenia I. Pe'nisson-Besnier De'partement de neurologie, center de re'fe'rence des maladies neuromusculaires, CHU d'Angers, 4, rue Larrey, 49933 Angers cedex 09, France

[14]By reversibly inhibiting the enzymatic hydrolysis of ACh in the synaptic cleft, anticholinesterase agents prolong the action of the neurotransmitter, thereby increasing the number of interactions with the remaining RACh.

[15] MYASTHENIA Myasthenia Gravis A. EL MIDAOUI, O. MESSOUAK, MF. BELAHSEN Neurology Department, CHU Hassan II, Fès, MOROCCO

[16] vidal.fr/medicaments/intratect-50-g-l-sol-p-perf-ait-225368.html#indesirable-effects

[17]Swiss Medical Journal - www.revmed.ch - May 9, 2007

18. Mekrani S, Brignol TN, Autoimmune myasthenia 10/ 2006. ISSN : 1769-1850.

19. Cambier J, Masson M et al. Abrèges neurologie 13th edition, ISBN: 978-2-294-71451-1. 2012. 509-516.

20. Ameri A, Timsit S, Guide pratique neurologie clinique. ISSN : 1248-5470.1997.162-172.

21. Oosterhuis.H, Myasthenia gravis. Edinburgh: Churchill Linvingstone, 1984

22. Mollaret P, Bastin R, Goulon M et al. Treatment by tracheostomy and artificial respiration in acute respiratory failure. In: Rapport au congrès français de médecine. Paris : Masson, 1959.

23. Simpson JA, Myasthenia gravis as an autoimmune disease: clinical aspects. Ann N Y Acad Sci 1966; 135: 506-516.

24. Engel AG, Santa T, Histometric analysis of the ultrastructure of the neuro muscular junction in myasthenia gravis and in the myasthenic syndrome. Ann N Y Acad Sci 1971 ; 183 : 46-63.

25. Fambrough D, Drachman D, Satyamurti S, Neuromuscular junction in myasthenia gravis: decreased Ach-R. Science 1973 ; 182 : 293-295.

26. Albuquerque EX, Rash JE et al. An electrophysiological and morphological

study of the neuromuscular junction in patients with MG. Exp Neurol 1976; 51: 536-563.

27. Lindstrom J, An assay for antibodies to human acetylcholine receptor in serum from patients with myasthenia gravis. Clin Immunol Immunopathol1977; 7: 36-43.

28. Carr AS, Cardwell CR, McCarron PO, McConville J, A systematic review of population based epidemiological studies in Myasthenia Gravis. BMC Neurol 2010;10:46.

29. Protocole National de Diagnostic et de Soins (PNDS), Autoimmune myasthenia, Centre de références de pathologie neuromusculaire Paris Est, July 2015.

30. Meriggioli MN, Sanders DB, Autoimmune myasthenia gravis: emerging clinical and biological heterogeneity. Lancet Neurol. 2009; 8 (5): 475-490.

31. Juel VC, Massey JM. Myasthenia gravis. Orphanet J Rare Dis, 2007; 2.

32. Hyung SL, Hye SL et cal. The Epidemiology of Myasthenia Gravis in Korea, Departments of Neurology and Biostatistics, Yonsei University College of Medicine, Seoul, Korea, Yonsei Med J 2016 Mar;57(2):419-425.

33. Masson C, Lecorre F, Boukriche Y. The peripheral acetylcholine receptor: physiology, pathophysiology applied to neuromuscular diseases and curarization. Réanimation. 2001 ; 10 (4) : 360-367.

34. JF Camps, D Eugéne et al. Neurosciences : tout le cours en fiches, 2013, EAN 978-2-10-058504-5, 88-109.

35. Lammens S, Hounfodji P, Krejci E, Plaud B. Physiology of the motor plate. In: Elsevier Editions. Congrès national d'anesthésie et de réanimation 2007.325-340.

36. Aurelie C. Assessing the needs of patients with myasthenia, particularly from the pharmacist's point of view. Pharmaceutical Sciences. 2013. <dumas-00840104>. http://dumas.ccsd.cnrs.fr/dumas-00840104.

37. Juel VC, Massey JM, Myasthenia gravis. Orphanet J Rare Dis, 2007; 2

38. Meriggioli MN, Sanders DB. Autoimmune myasthenia gravis: emerging clinical and biological heterogeneity. Lancet Neurol. 2009 ; 8 (5) : 475-490.

39. Mekrani S, Brignol TN. Autoimmune myasthenia, Savoir et comprendre. AFM. 2006.

40. Herson S, Tranchant C. Myasthenia gravis. Encyclopédie Orphanet Grand Public. 2009. www.orpha.net/data/patho/Pub/fr/MyasthenieAcquise- FRfrPub667v01.pdf consulted online on 14/06/2012.

41. Goldenberg WD, Shah AK. Myasthenia Gravis. Medscapereference. http://emedicine.medscape.com/article/1171206-overview#showall last accessed 10/03/2013.

42. H Déchy, B Wechsler, P Hausfater et al, Atteintes neurologiques au cours des maladies systémiques 72-77.

43. ChaupLannaz G, Vial C, Electrodiagnosis of junctional diseases. neuromuscular, rev.Neural, 2000, 156 :76-81.

44. Morel E, Raimond F, Goulon-Goëau C, Berrih S et al. Le dosage des anticrécepteurs de l'acétylcholine dans la myasthénie. Presse Méd 1982; 11: 1849- 1854.

45. Berrih-Aknin S, Morel E, Raimond F et al. The role of the thymus in myasthenia gravis. Immunohistological and immunological studies in 115 cases. AnnN Y Acad Sci 1987 ; 505 : 50-70.

46. Goulon-Goëau C. Contribution personnelle au dosage des anticrécepteurs de l'acétylcholine dans la myasthénie et étude de leur corrélation avec l'évolution clinique. [thesis], Paris, 1982.

47. Vincent A, Newsom-Davis J. Acetylcholine receptor antibody as a diagnostic test for myasthenia gravis. J NeurolNeurosurgPsychiatry 1985; 48: 1246-1252.

48. Drachman DB. Myasthenia gravis. NEnglJMed1994;330: 1797-1810.

49. David C, Paul M, François des gands champs, guide de 1ers ordonnances, December 2010, 356-360.

50 Gold R, Hohlfeld R, Toyka KV. Progress in the treatment of myasthenia gravis. Ther Adv Neurol Disord. 2008; 1 (2): 36-51.

51. Jani-Acsadi A, Lisak RP. Myasthenic crisis: Guidelines for prevention and treatment. J Neurol Sci. 2007; 261 (1-2): 127-133.

52. Chaudhuri A, Behan PO. Myasthenic crisis. Q J Med. 2009; 102:97-107.

53. Newsom-Davis J, Beeson D, Myasthenia gravis and myasthenic syndrome: autoimmune and genetic desorders. In: G. Karpati, D. hilton-Jones, RC.Griggs, disorders of volentary muscles, Cambridge, cambridge university press,2001: 600-677.

54. Bever CT, Aquino A, Penn AS, Lovelace RE, Rowland LP. Prognosis of ocular myasthenia. Ann Neurol 1983; 14: 516-519.

55. Mosman S, Vincent A, Newson-Davis J. Myasthenia gravis without acetylcholine-receptor antibody :adistinct disease entity. Lancet 1986; 1: 116-119.

56. Willcox N, Schluep M, Ritter MA, Newsom-Davis J. The thymus in seronegative myasthenia gravis patients. J Neurol 1991; 238: 256-261.

57. SD Weatherbee, KV Anderson, LA Niswander, LDL-receptor-related protein 4 is crucial for formation of the neuromuscular junction, Development 133 (2006) 4993-5000.

58. N Kim, AL Stiegler, TO Cameron, PT Hallock, AM Gomez et al. Lrp4 is a receptor for Agrin and forms a complex with MuSK, Cell 135 (2008) 334-342.

59. B Zhang, S Luo, Q Wang, et al, LRP4 serves as a coreceptor of agrin, Neuron 60 (2008) 285-297.

60. O Higuchi, J Hamuro, M Motomura, Y Yamanashi, Autoantibodies to lowdensity lipoprotein receptor-related protein 4 in myasthenia gravis, Ann. Neurol. 69 (2011) 418-422.

61. A Pevzner, B Schoser, K Peters, NC Cosma et al, Anti-LRP4 autoantibodies in AChR- and MuSK-antibody-negative myasthenia gravis, J. Neurol. 259 (2012) 427- 435.

62. David C, Paul M, François des gands champs, guide de 1ers ordonnances, December 2010, 356-360.

63. Advances in autoimmune myasthenia June 2016, editorial: myoinfo information department on neuromuscular diseases, AFM-Téléthon, Evry.

64. Pénission-Besnier I. Treatment of autoimmune myasthenia. Review neurology. 2010 ; 166 : 400-405.

65. Dorosz P. Guide pratique des médicaments Dorosz 2010. 29th ed: Maloine; 2009.

66. Goulon-Goeau C et Gajdos P. Myasthenia and myasthenic syndromes. Encycl Méd Chir (Editions Scientifiques et Médicales Elsevier SAS, Paris, all rights reserved), Neurologie, 17-172-B-10, 2002, 14 p.

67. Gilchrist JM. Myasthenia gravis. Medical update for psychiatrists. 1998; 3 (4):113-118.

68. ANSM. Répertoire des spécialités pharmaceutiques. http://agenceprd. ansm.sante.fr/php/ecodex/index.php , last consulted December 2012.

69. Vidal dictionary. 2011. ISBN : 978-2-85091-189-9.

70 Warmolts JR, Engel WK. Benefits from alternate-day prednisone in myasthenia gravis. N Engl J Med 1972 ; 286 : 17-20.

71. Delwaide PJ, Salmon J, van Cauwenberger H. First treatment trials of myasthenia by azathioprine. Acta Neurol Belg1967; 67: 701-712.

72. Johns TR. Long-term corticosteroid treatment of myasthenia gravis. Ann N Y Acad Sci 1987; 505: 568-583.

73. Pascuzzi RM, Coslett HB, Johns TR. Long-term corticosteroid treatment of myasthenia gravis: report of116patients. Ann Neurol 1984 ; 15 : 291-298.

74. Sanders DS, Howard JJ, Johns TR, CampaJF. High dose daily prednisone in the treatment of myasthenia gravis. In: Plasmapheresis and the immunobiology of myasthenia gravis. Boston : Houghton, Mifflin Pubfishers, 1979 : 289-306.

75. Sghirlanzoni A, Peluchetti D, Mantegazza R, Fiacchino F, Cornelio F. Myasthenia gravis: prolonged treatment with steroids. Neurology 1984; 34: 170-174.

76. Turner C. A Review of myasthenia gravis: Pathogenesis, clinical features and treatment. Currentanaesthesia and critical care. 2007; 18 (1):15-23.

77. Drug interactions. Understanding and deciding. La Revue Prescrire.
2011 ; 31 (338) Suppl.

78. Garcia-Carrasco M, Escarcega RO et al. Therapeutic options in autoimmune myasthenia gravis. AutoimmunRev. 2007; 6:373-378.

79. Goulon M, Gadjos PH, Estournet B. Treatment of myasthenia by plasma exchange and immunosuppressants. In: Hémoperfusion. Échanges plasmatiques en réanimation. Paris: Expansion Scientifique Française, 1981: 325-338.

80. Olarte MR, Schoenfeldt RS, Penn AS, Lovelace RE, Rowland LP. Effects of plasmapheresis in myasthenia gravis 1978- 1980. Ann N Y Acad Sci 1981 ; 377 :725-728.

81 Masson et al, 2001.

82.Camps et al . 2013

83 Nazinigouba et al, 2011

84.Svahn et al . 2018

85.Krieff, 2014

86.Benchekroun, 2016

87 Juel and Massey, 2007.

88.Gajdos, 2005.

89.Chenevier et al. 2011.

90.Mantegazza et al. 2018.

91.Koneczny and Herbst, 2019.

92.Eymard, 2009.

93 Thanvi and Lo TCN, 2004.

94.Gilhus et al . 2016

95.Catar et al . 2017

96.Bensafi et al., 2015

97.Niks et al . 2008

98.Rivner et al., 2018

99.Morren and Li, 2018

100.Berrih-Aknin and Le panse ,2014

101.Koneczny and Herbst, 2019).

102 Pevzner et al. 2012

103.Yan et al . 2018

104 Higuchi et al., 2011

105. Wirtz PW, Nijnuis MG, Sotodeh M et al. The epidemiology of myasthenia gravis, Lambert-Eaton myasthenic syndrome and their associated tumoursin the northern part of the province of South Holland. J Neurol 2003; 250: 698-701.

106.Oosterhuis H.J.G.H, Myasthenia gravis, Groningen neurological press 1997, p252.

107.Vincent et al., 2008

108 Leite et al. 2008

109 Le Pance et al, 2008

110.Berrih-Aknin and Le Pance, 2014).

111 Leite et al.,2005

112 Scarpino et al. 2007

113.Le Panse R, Cizeron-Clairac G et al. Regulatory and pathogenic mechanisms in human autoimmune myasthenia gravis. Ann N YAcadSci. 2008; 1132: 135-142.

114 El Midaoui et al., 2010

115 Miyazawa et al, 2003

116.Sudhof, 1999

117 Lammens et al. 2007

118.Benchekroun, 2016

119. NIH Consensus Conference. The utility of therapeutic plasmapheresis for neurological disorders. JAMA 1986; 256: 1333-1337.

120 Arsura E, Brunner NG, Namba T, Grob D. High-dose intravenous methyl prednisolone in myasthenia gravis. Arch Neurol 1985; 42: 1149-1153.

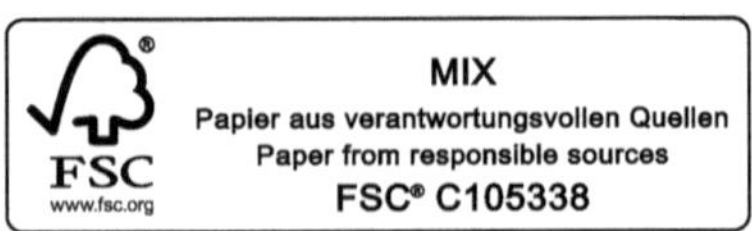

Printed by Books on Demand GmbH, Norderstedt / Germany